HEAL BREAST CANCER NATURALLY

7 ESSENTIAL STEPS TO BEATING BREAST CANCER

DR. VÉRONIQUE DESAULNIERS

DISCLAIMER

The information presented in this book is for educational and informational purposes only. It is not intended to be a substitute for proper diagnosis and treatment by a licensed professional. If you have any questions about whether the information and advice presented in this book is suitable for you, please check with your trusted physician or health care provider. It is your responsibility to discern what information provided is useful for your health and to use this guide in appropriate and common sense ways.

The publisher has put forth its best efforts in preparing and arranging this book. The information provided herein by the author is provided 'as is' and you read and use this information at your own risk. The publisher and author disclaim any liabilities for any loss of profit or commercial or personal damages resulting from the use of the information contained in this eBook.

Cambria font used with permission from Microsoft.

Edited by: Sherrie Dolby

http://www.amazon.com/Sherrie-Dolby/e/B009Y1Z3BM/

ISBN: 978-1-63161-991-5

Published by TCK Publishing

www.TCKPublishing.com

CONTENTS

Disclaimer and Waiver

Read This FIRST!

I am **not** a medical doctor, dentist, oncologist, or breast specialist and I do **not** represent myself as one. First and foremost, I am a woman who personally experienced Breast Cancer. I literally stared Breast Cancer in the face and conquered it. I am a licensed Doctor of Chiropractic with over 35 years of experience in the Wellness Industry. My passion is empowering women about an evidence-based way of supporting and healing the body.

Natural Medicine, holistic medicine, or whatever you wish to call it, has been scientifically validated for years. I encourage you to take the time to review the hyperlinks and references that I have cited. Many of the links will take you to the United States Library of Medicine, www.pubmed.gov, a service of the National Institute of Health, paid for by your tax dollars.

In the search bar, type in a natural substance and Breast Cancer and you will see hundreds of studies validating the effect of that substance on Breast Cancer. For example, type in "selenium and Breast Cancer" and over 375 studies will pop up, proving the positive effect that selenium has on Breast Cancer patients and how selenium reduces Breast Cancer metastasis. You will see study after study that validates the power of Natural Medicine.

I did not use traditional diagnostic ways to 'confirm' that I had Breast Cancer. I chose not to have my breasts radiated and compressed, nor did I want to have a biopsy that could potentially spread the cancer. I was not interested in a 'label' or a 'stage'. To me, cancer was cancer, and I had to get to the CAUSE of what allowed it to develop in the first place.

For some of you, the methods that I chose to detect and heal the Breast Cancer may seem outrageous, unscientific, and impossible. The methodologies that I used and describe in this book are not for everyone.

The information presented in this book has **not** been approved by the FDA, AMA, or any Federal or State agency. This book is for educational purposes only and is **not** intended, nor should it be used, as a substitute for medical advice. Consult a licensed, qualified medical physician for any issues concerning your health. Your physician should be aware of all your medical conditions as well as any medications and nutritional supplements you are taking. Search for a doctor that will support you with your goals of prevention or of healing. Anyone who wishes to embark on a healing journey involving any dietary or lifestyle changes accepts full responsibility for their decision.

Breast Cancer Conqueror, LLC as well as Dr. Véronique Desaulniers-Chomniak are **not** responsible for any decisions you make as a result of reading the information in this book. If you wish to embark on a healing program, work under the supervision of a licensed health care practitioner who has had success in your area of concern. The information in this book is not a substitute for professional medical advice. The contents of this book may be considered controversial by the traditional medical community.

Neither the author, editor, nor publisher will be responsible for damages arising out of or in connection with the use of this book. The information in this book provides content related to topics about health issues. As such, reading this book and the use of this book implies your acceptance of this disclaimer and waiver.

FOREWORD

What you are holding in your hand or reading on your computer screen is a very valuable resource. You probably are not as aware as I am how valuable this is to you. Having written 3 books on natural cancer healing and helping about 5,000 people in 66 countries heal themselves of cancer, I think I'm qualified to advise you.

Please sit down, relax, and read this book. Dr. V is a unique resource. She has healed herself of breast cancer and helped thousands of others heal before and after her own experience with her knowledge. She is a qualified medical professional and a cancer survivor. I am neither. I'm just a guy whose wife was killed by the cancer doctors 20 years ago and who has been inspired by that experience to help lots of other people avoid my late wife's fate. But I'm not the medical professional or cancer survivor that Dr. V is, so I'm urging you to pay attention to what she has to tell you.

In my 16 years of helping cancer patients, they have taught me why people get cancer and what they do to heal themselves of it – permanently. Dr. V knows this. We agree on the approach to cancer that works. This book gives you the information you need to avoid cancer if you haven't experienced it yet and to heal it permanently if you have.

The title suggests that this information is confined to breast cancer. Forget that. My experience is that 'cancer is cancer'. Regardless of its location, type, stage, etc., it is the same thing. Dr. V understands this. It is simply a symptom of an imbalance in your body – caused by something. It is not a random physical event. If you have a cancer diagnosis, it is simply a result of things that have happened to you over the years preceding it. These include – almost always in my experience – stressful and emotional experiences, dental toxins, and what we put in our mouths.

Yes, the cancer is almost always caused by 'triggers' that are the result of our lifestyle choices. There are other causes – what ill-informed dentists do to our teeth and jaws, what ill-informed doctors do to our bodies, for example. However, almost always one of the reasons cancer becomes diagnosable is because of what we've chosen to eat and drink and smoke throughout our lives. Our environment – particularly difficult relationships with other people – is almost always involved as well.

The good news is that we can almost always correct and reverse these causes once we understand them. Dr. V has given you a great book here to help you do exactly that. Of course, when you elect to trust the cancer doctors to treat you, you make that outcome much harder. There is no treatment offered by cancer doctors that helps cancer to heal. It all makes your situation worse.

Having worked with thousands of people, most of whom have submitted to some conventional 'cut, burn, poison' treatment, I know that it is never time to give up. Any cancer condition can be reversed. Is it possible to get to the 'point of no return'? Sure. But this is usually because of insistence on the part of the cancer patient to continue subjecting themselves to conventional cancer treatment instead of backing off from that treatment and taking charge of their own health care.

You are in a position now to take complete charge of your prevention or healing and succeed at avoiding or overcoming cancer. This book will give you the ammunition and knowledge you need. Use it and enjoy new, wonderful health. It's your right, and Dr. V has given you what you need to claim it.

Bill Henderson, Cancer Coach

Author, *Cure Your Cancer, How to Cure Almost Any Cancer At Home For $5.15 A Day* and *Cancer-Free, Your Guide to Gentle, Non-toxic Healing* **www.Beating-Cancer-Gently.com**

Testimonials

"Dr. V. was the first person that I thought about when I was diagnosed with breast cancer. I called her even before I told my family. From our first consultation, I felt her care and compassion. I felt supported and understood. Thank you Dr. V."

F.L. Quebec, Canada

"When I was diagnosed with Breast Cancer I felt scared, confused, and alone. Dr. V. gave me the knowledge and information I needed. She understands the emotional side of breast cancer, having been there herself. She has now become a trusted friend."

D.R. Australia

"As a Breast Cancer survivor, the information about the 7 essentials has been priceless! The information that Dr. V. has shared with me has led me to a healthier lifestyle. I support and continue to enjoy our relationship with all the positive feedback I have gained."

MJ M, Florida

"Thank you Dr. V. for being the 'calm' in my shaken world... Your gentle care and wisdom has gone far to encourage me through my Breast Cancer recovery journey! I am blessed by your ministry to help others."

S. L. California

"After being diagnosed with Breast Cancer, I began Dr. V's program. Three months later, the lump was gone and so were the cancer cells. I was able to give my beautiful baby the precious gift of breastfeeding."

T.R., Illinois

"Dr. V. is happy to answer any questions and help a woman go through such a hard period as Breast Cancer. I am now cancer free."

L.M. Slovakia

"Dr. V. picked me up in my time of need and gently laid out an action plan. She reminded me that we have choices. Because of Dr. V, I will rally through this (Breast Cancer) and become even more whole!"

Dr. J.A. Georgia

"I was told to get my affairs in order and that I had 4 months to live. After 6 months, there were minimal cancer cells, and I was able to return to work. Doctors were shocked at my recovery. Working with Dr. V. has given me a life to fight for."

W.M. Illinois

"Dr. V exhibited a high level of personal concern for me and attentively listened as I explained my health concerns. This continued on beyond our initial consultation, and I found her to be a very kind and caring individual with a vast array of knowledge. She showed to me a genuine interest in my welfare, and I am blessed to be in her care."

P.B. Florida

"I am so grateful to be working with Dr. V. She is excellent with providing information and sharing the research that goes with it. I also appreciate that she provides options for us and leaves us to decide what is best, all in a professional, caring, and supportive manner."

L. C. California

"Professional, knowledgeable, passionate, and caring. Those words best describe Dr. V. I have known her for over 20 years, and her results have been remarkable."

Dr. D.C., MD, Florida

"Having a friend and/or coach to help you through any difficult time is essential. I consider myself a step ahead having her guidance and expertise available to me."

Dr. K.L. Georgia

"Dr. V's personal attention and concern gave me a positive outlook for the future. The natural alternative methods enhanced my health tremendously without any negative side-effects. I am forever grateful."

R.P. Illinois

"I have known Dr. V for over 30 years and highly recommend her services as a coach and doctor for anyone that is tired of medical doctors treating symptoms and not getting to the cause. Her knowledge and caring heart are priceless."

D.C. Georgia

"I have been under Dr. V's care for 25 years and have never been disappointed. I always get good results with her recommendations. When I first met her she was kind, compassionate, and understanding and to this day, she still remains true to those endearing qualities."

C.D. Georgia

"Dr. V is professional yet nurturing. I have witnessed amazing results."

G.D. Manitoba, Canada

Dedication and Inspiration

To Lucille and Achilles, who were the best parents that they could possibly be. Life was not easy for you. Ironically, your pain and sorrow became the inspiration to live my life to the fullest.

Dad, 'le Père', I wish I understood cancer back then like I do now. You slipped away so quickly because of the pancreatic cancer. But before you did, you told me you loved me. Thank you.

Mum, 'la Mère', you allowed me to teach you about healing Breast Cancer naturally. That was a very proud moment for me. I wish I could have healed your heart, both literally and figuratively. I am thankful that I was able to hold your hand all night before you slipped away so quietly the next morning.

To my children, Janique, Chantale, and Justin 'Jahret', the joys of my life. From the moment I held you in my arms after your home births, I knew that there was an unbreakable bond that sealed our lives forever. You love me with such heart and depth, and you love each other just the same. I am truly a blessed woman to have experienced the joys of motherhood with you.

To my husband Brian, my 'Muzz', who is my soul mate. With all my heart, I believed I would eventually find you, and I did. You have loved me like no other and have stood by me like no other. You reminded me how beautiful life really is, and you taught me to laugh once again. Je t'aime de tout mon coeur!

The Beginning

"Miracles come in moments. Be ready and willing."

~

Dr. Wayne Dyer

If you look back on your life, there are usually some pretty defining moments that make you go, "AHA." These moments change the course of your life and lead you down a totally different path than what you may have originally planned for your future.

I was a shy, emotionally wounded, French Canadian girl who grew up in a small French community and had plans to become a veterinarian and save wounded and stray animals. I loved animals and was very attracted to them because of the unconditional love that they so generously gave. I was going to make a difference in the world and become a 'Daktari', a veterinarian in Africa (remember that TV series?).

But one early Saturday morning, sitting on the side of the bed, I was introduced to the science, art, and philosophy of Chiropractic by my cousin and BFF, Jocelyne.

Jocelyne invited me to attend a 'health lecture' hosted by a new, up and coming Chiropractor, Dr. Gil. I will never forget the feeling of sitting in that chair and listening to the Universal truths that he was discussing.

"Health is your birth right. Follow specific laws, and your body can heal and recover. Put good things IN your body and your health will reflect that. Your Nerve System is the master computer of your body and a subluxated spine can impede the transmission of life-promoting energy to your organs and cells."

It was a defining moment for me.

My childhood was not the easiest of childhoods. The stress of alcoholic parents, sexual abuse from a convicted pedophile neighbor, and emotional neglect were all part of my childhood. That little girl felt sadness, stress, fear, and loneliness. I was never allowed to be a carefree, fun-loving child since I was always worried about my parents and 'taking care of them'. I love and have forgiven my parents since I know they did the best they knew how, with the information they had. They themselves were wounded children, so they had weak parenting and nurturing skills.

Growing up in the 50s and 60s in south-central Canada, our meals consisted of a lot of canned foods, meats, white breads, and lots of sugar. Rarely was there any fresh produce on the table, other than an occasional salad in the summer. I suffered constantly with digestive upsets, nervous stomach, chronic constipation, moving my bowels once per week in a good week, and chronic headaches. WOW! How did I survive?

Thus, when I heard the positive message of hope with Chiropractic and healthy living, I was focused on sharing this message with others. I knew at that moment that I wanted to bring wellness to the world. At the tender age of 16, I fell in love with herbal teas, healthier food, and exercise.

On a physical level, my life was improving and I was feeling better, but I had not broken free from the dysfunctional patterns and learned behaviors of alcoholism and depression. I went through some very traumatic, life-changing events as a young adult and found myself feeling very dark and depressed.

Then one fateful day, my Chiropractor called me and invited me to go for coffee after my appointment with him. Another defining moment....

He knew what I had experienced in the last few months, (remember that I lived in a small community) and wanted to reach out to me. Rather than being judgmental and critical of my life choices, he recognized my potential and my inner beauty. I will never forget his words,

"You are young, bright, and beautiful. You love Chiropractic and what it stands for. You have a very bright future ahead of you."

As he said those words, he reached into his lapel pocket and handed me an application to Life College in Marietta, Georgia. When I reached over the table and held that application in my hand, I felt an electric spark travel throughout my body. I had immediate visions of a happier and healthier life.

I had NO idea how all this was going to happen, but I pushed forward. How could it be possible for a shy French Canadian, inexperienced young woman to move to a foreign country and become a doctor? The odds seemed to be against me, but my determination and desire made it happen. I am forever grateful for my parents and the financial support that they provided for me to live my dream.

March 7, 1977, I was on a plane to Atlanta, GA. My life would never be the same.

As I attended Life College, my eyes were opened to the power of the body's capacity to heal. I was introduced to every type of diet and lifestyle imaginable; everything from macrobiotics, vegetarianism, veganism, cotton only clothes, energy healing, magnets, and massage. This whole new world of 'healthy lifestyles' created several healing crises and detox periods. I was expelling the accumulation of a lifetime of toxic foods and habits. I was cleaning physically, emotionally, and spiritually.

In 1980, I opened my doors as a licensed Chiropractor, excited about bringing this message of health and hope to as many people as possible. I had the privilege of touching the lives of thousands of people. As my patients improved their diets, supplemented with specific herbs and vitamins, I was witnessing amazing results with all kinds of health issues. My practice was thriving and I was healing.

Then, in 1983, another life-changing event: my father Achilles was diagnosed with pancreatic cancer. He was given no hope, no encouragement, and was sent home to die, which he did in 6 weeks. I will never forget my feelings of hopelessness and frustration.

"Surely there is something that can be done to heal cancer. I knew some of my patients had done it and so could my father."

Life before the Internet meant that we had to go to the library, read books, and get on the phone to make connections with people. As I dug deeper, I was reading accounts of specific herbs and protocols that reversed cancers of all types. I got on the phone and talked to alternative cancer doctors who were seeing amazing results with their cancer patients. But, unfortunately for my father, it was too late.

That event opened up the 'cancer door' for me. It gave me a better understanding of how and why so many of my aunts and uncles had died of cancer. I studied hard and became certified in bio-energetic testing, homeopathy, and herbal medicines. I was now understanding health and healing on a whole new level.

I began to attract patients with very challenging health issues. As I taught the principles of natural medicine, my patients were turning their health around.

It was so heartwarming to see lives transformed as their physical problems disappeared and they could now enjoy life with a whole new appreciation.

Fast forward 10 years, and my mother was diagnosed with Breast Cancer. She had a lumpectomy and so much radiation that her breast was red hot and hard as a brick until the day she died. She did not want to do chemo, so she came to visit her daughter, Dr. V., to try a more natural and gentler approach to healing. I was so proud of my mom and how she religiously took her drops and herbs. She never had an issue with cancer again.

Then came another defining moment. One morning in April of 2004, I was in the shower getting ready for another fulfilling day at the office, when I noticed a hard marble-like lump in my left breast. I kept feeling it from every angle, telling myself that it was nothing, but the burning pit in my stomach and in my chest told me otherwise.

I consulted with an MD friend of mine whom I will call Dr. Dan. Dr. Dan was having tremendous success with cancer patients without the use of toxic therapies. Bio-energetic testing confirmed it was Breast Cancer. Some of you may be thinking,

"No blood work? No official name? No biopsy? How did you know you really had cancer?"

Keep reading, and you will understand.

By now I had been in practice for 24 years, and I had witnessed the unpleasant effects of the traditional cancer conveyor-belt system: cut, poison, and burn. If the body was strong enough, it could on occasion survive the treatments, but not without chronic and life-changing side effects.

On the flip side, I also witnessed how supportive, natural therapies strengthened the body's immune system and weakened cancer cells, so there was no question or second guessing what my path would be. I had full confidence in my body's ability to heal.

I have to admit that at first I really didn't believe that this lump was cancer. I was pretty much in denial. After all, how could Dr. V develop Breast Cancer? I ate organic before organic was in style, I had home births, breast fed all 3 children for 18 months each, I exercised regularly, I was under Chiropractic care, and I had a regular regime of supplements and herbs, including wheat grass. I kept asking questions and praying so I could understand what I was going to learn from this event. What was this going to teach me?

In the early years of my practice, I had seen a few cancer patients use a 'black salve' to physically remove, and accelerate the extraction, of a tumor from their body. I was in shock and disbelief when I first learned about this. I saw the tumor in a jar and the hole in their body where the tumor used to be. It was incredible! But as I began to understand the bio-chemical makeup of the salve, it made total sense.

The salve consisted of blood root, zinc chloride, galangal, and a few other herbs and oils. Blood Root is a perennial that has a compound in it called Sanguinarine. Sanguinarine causes cancer cells to die, without affecting healthy cells. How is that for a healing form of 'herbal chemo'! This is simply another example of selective toxicity found in Nature – destroying unhealthy cells without harming healthy ones.

I decided that I would apply that salve so I flipped through magazines and several journals and lo and behold, I found a small ad for black salve. I ordered it and decided to see what would happen. Big mistake! I went into this experience blindly and totally unprepared. I was still in denial about actually having a tumor in my breast, so I took the salve experience pretty lightly until Day 4.

Day 4 got my attention. The salve was creating a hole in my breast, and it burned like fire as it did! What was happening? I freaked out and panicked a little. I called the manufacturer of the salve and wanted an explanation and support. He was very nonchalant about it, did not give me clear direction, or what to expect in the future.

"Just keep applying it, and it will eventually fall out. Since the lump reacted, *there is cancer in the breast*. Blood root will not react or touch healthy cells. If the lump was benign, there would have been no reaction."

Maybe he was afraid of the legal ramifications and was being careful about what he was telling me on the phone. I don't know. All I know is that I felt very scared and very alone. After he hung up, I sat on the bathroom floor, clutching the phone, and sobbed uncontrollably for an hour. This really was Breast Cancer!

Another defining moment. It's time to take this seriously. I called my friend Dr. Dan and sent him pictures. He confirmed. Yes, definitely Breast Cancer.

I continued to apply the salve everyday as instructed. I took a barrage of immune boosting supplements, homeopathics, and herbal botanicals. The pain reminded me of labor pains, only this time I was birthing a tumor. By week three the hole had developed into a huge crater that was erupting from my skin. The burning pain was the most excruciating pain I've ever experienced. As the edges started to separate, I could see 'inside' my breast! YIKES!! How strange was that?! As the scab or eschar continued to separate, the pain decreased. Hallelujah!

Then one morning as I was changing the bandage, I could tell that the eschar or scab was simply hanging on by a thread. I leaned over and it fell out of my breast. I will never forget that moment-relief-disbelief-fear and confusion all wrapped into one. I was staring at this tumor that used to be in my breast and now it was sitting on a tissue. Now what?

I was instructed by Dr. Dan to spray the wound with hydrogen peroxide and lavender oil and to keep it well bandaged. I examined the crater in my breast and there was a noticeable black, dark spot. It almost reminded me of a reptilian eye winking at me. What the heck was that?

More pictures sent to Dr. Dan. Good news, bad news. Good news was the edges were clean and the big tumor was gone. Bad news was there was still some residual unhealthy tissue in the breast.

My heart sank and my knees weakened. What? After all that? I had two choices:

A - Reapply the salve in the hole and on the residual tumor or...

B - Continue to spray and bandage and let the wound heal up. Definitely keep working on the internal protocol with nutrition, herbs, and homeopathy.

So for the next two years, I followed a somewhat regimented program of clean, healthy, organic living. Life was full and busy and my personal experience seemed to attract more and more women looking for alternative methods to heal their bodies.

Another defining moment: in 2005, I discovered Thermography. I had my first Thermogram done, and there was a big hot spot in my left breast indicating inflammation and angiogenesis (the formation of new blood vessels). My staff and I began to incorporate digital Thermographic imaging and other powerful tools to help monitor the physiology of the body. This camera was a great aid in confirming physiological progress with women who had challenges with their breasts and overall health. I kept monitoring my breasts with thermography and bio-energetic testing.

Unfortunately, things did not progress the way I expected and anticipated. **It was obvious that there was some serious angiogenesis (blood flow feeding a tumor) developing. The inflamed area had grown in size.**

After several consultations with doctors and a Ph.D. familiar with this process, I decided to extract the tumor once again with the use of the black salve. The 2004 "I will never do this again" pain was in the distant past. This time, however, I was better prepared.

I had found a company that specialized in black salve and natural cancer protocols. I tested the salve and the supplements bio-energetically, and they tested very well on myself and most patients. The company had an excellent support system and was consistently having success with various cancers.

The second application of the salve from beginning to end lasted about four weeks. It was fast and furious. When the eschar released and fell off, the wound was clean and there was no 'reptilian eye' winking at me. Victory at last! I had conquered Breast Cancer naturally.

As I began sharing my story and experience with other women, they would often ask me,

"If you were so healthy and doing all the right things, why did you STILL get cancer?"

Excellent question and one that I asked myself a gazillion times. But you know the saying, 'Ask and you shall receive'? I became the student and opened my heart and mind, and the answers started coming, and they are still coming to this day.

Here are just a few more AHA moments that changed my life and defined the basis for The 7 Essentials:

- Electrical pollution and EMF's cause DNA damage and impair the Immune System.
- Emotional trauma and poorly managed stress creates hormonal changes that impair your body's ability to heal.
- Improper methylation and estrogen metabolism cause DNA damage and can lead to cancer and a number of other diseases.
- Lack of proper sleep can silence cancer-protective genes.
- Low iodine levels and a sluggish thyroid increase the risk of Breast Cancer.
- There are specific nutrients that can turn on cancer-protective genes.

The information in this book is a culmination of over 35 years of personal and professional experience with natural medicines. I decided to write this book because I wanted to impart hope to women that are faced with the diagnosis of Breast Cancer. I know what it feels like to be faced with the maze of Internet information and not know which direction to go or even where to start.

I know what it feels like to be scared and to experience pain and doubt.

While I was on my healing journey, one typical morning, I walked by the kitchen table and picked up a magazine that caught my attention. There was an article about a man named Sean Stephenson who was afflicted with osteogenesis imperfecti, a bone disease that causes the bones to be so brittle that they shatter and break. This 3 foot motivational speaker traveled the world to share his story and move people to appreciate all the gifts they had in their everyday lives.

He related that when he was a child, there was a significant event that changed his life forever. After fracturing another bone in one of his legs, simply from playing outside in the yard, he was crying, frustrated, mad, and feeling sorry for himself. His mother looked at him and said, ***"Is this going to be a gift or is this going to a burden? You get to choose."***

Now as fascinating as that story was, it was clear that the message was meant for me and what I was experiencing. Those words were exactly what I needed to read at that very moment. I had a choice. I could look at my experience with cancer as a burden or I could choose to appreciate it as a gift.

I chose to look at it as a gift, and I ask you to do the same. That can be challenging at times, especially if you are feeling low emotionally and physically. Pray for insight and guidance so that you grow emotionally and spiritually as you heal your physical body.

The 7 Essentials came as a result of years of research and soul-searching. It is a step-by-step guide that will hold your hand through the process of preventing Breast Cancer or any type of disease for that matter. It will also serve as a reference for you as you embark on your healing journey with Breast Cancer. It will open doors for you. It will teach you.

You will have your highs and lows but you will also have your own glorious AHA moments when it all seems to come together. Celebrate when you make progress. Celebrate and be grateful for the positive changes that are occurring.

Can I make the claim that you will be cancer-free if you follow The 7 Essentials? Legally and ethically, I can't. Sadly, some people die even though they seem to have done everything right. Others don't apply half the principles, and they breeze through their cancer journey without much problem.

Take responsibility for your health. Make informed decisions.

CANCER CANNOT GROW IN A HEALTHY BODY

Your goal is to become healthy on every level, physically, mentally, emotionally, and spiritually.

If you have been diagnosed with Breast Cancer, or any other disease, there is something out of balance in your body. It may be your emotions which are suppressing your Immune System. It may be toxicity levels, acidity, lifestyle, or a combination of many things. Be brutally honest with yourself and take a measure of responsibility by making necessary changes.

You are not alone on this journey. There are hundreds of thousands of people that have successfully healed cancer with the use of evidence-based natural medicine. I'm simply asking you to think about your disease as a process, just as your healing will be a process. You did not 'get cancer' and then became sick. You were already sick and THEN you developed cancer. Be open to new ideas and stare cancer in the face, with less fear and more determination. Trust the process. Trust your body's ability to heal.

My vision for this book is that every person who holds the physical book in their hands or whose eyes gaze on the electronic version of this book has an AHA moment in some way. I pray this book serves as a successful guide for you so you never have to fear cancer again.

I've attempted to present many scientifically based facts in order for you to build confidence in this method of healing.

It was important for me that you understood that this information is not 'new age' fluff, but it is based on sound principles and scientific studies.

It would be virtually impossible to discuss all the various diets and the hundreds of protocols that have worked for many, since there is no cookie-cutter, one-size-fits-all method.

I have witnessed how our bodies have the miraculous power to heal and restore health, even in the face of the most serious and dire circumstances. Tens of thousands of women around the world have chosen to heal their bodies naturally. Many were initially coerced and intimidated into going down traditional toxic paths, only to wake up one day, realizing that the 'treatment' designed to 'kill the cancer' was also killing them.

Embarking on a healing journey is not just about learning the facts, having the proof, and following the protocols. It is about opening up your heart to growth, clearing your mind of past programming, and allowing the 'true you' to shine through. Often times, the major healing we have to do is found between our ears. Erroneous beliefs that have kept you captive most of your life can be changed into positive, supportive thought patterns.

Healing is like a metamorphosis and a transformation so that going forward you live your life from a greater consciousness and appreciation for every sunrise, every breath, and every heartbeat.

Many blessings to you and your family as you journey on your road to vibrant health!

Naturally,

Dr. V

CHAPTER 1

WHY DO I HAVE BREAST CANCER?

"The future is not something we enter…
The future is something we create."

~

Leonard I. Sweet

MORE THAN HALF OF ALL CANCERS ARE PREVENTABLE

Breast Cancer is not one 'disease', but it is an accumulation of many illnesses and weaknesses in the body. We live in an environmentally complex world inundated with foreign chemicals that assault our body every day. We may have chronic low-grade bacterial, fungal, or viral infections that are weakening and stressing our Immune system on a daily basis.

We are also exposed to the insidious effect of electro pollution and EMFs, while we're racing through life trying to 'get it all done'. Poor quality food, lack of sleep, and chronic stress is the formula for creating disease in the body. If you're reading this book, you're probably ready to take responsibility for your health and you realize that preventing and healing Breast Cancer goes beyond being a victim of your genes. It is about taking responsibility for your health and discovering what allowed the cancer to develop in the first place.

In the 1940's, your chances of developing Breast Cancer were 1:40. Now, 1:8 women will develop Breast Cancer in their lifetime. If you are not a Breast Cancer statistic, you then have a 1:3 chance to develop some other type of cancer in your lifetime. In February of 2014, the World Health Organization made a statement that there is an imminent global cancer disaster that will cause cancer cases to surge 57% in the next 20 years[1].

Scientists have come to the conclusion that more than half of all cancers can be prevented through lifestyle changes and healthier habits[2]. According to the University Of Columbia School Of Public Health, "95% of all cancer is due to diet and the accumulation of toxins."

Believe it or not, an article in the American Association of Pharmaceutical Scientists stated that

"Cancer is a preventable disease that requires major lifestyle changes. Only 5 - 10% of all cancer cases can be attributed to genetic defects, whereas the remaining 90-95% have their roots in the environment and lifestyle."[3]

When we look at these statements, it builds confidence that we can have significant control over our health and Breast Cancer outcomes. Preventing and healing Breast Cancer comes with taking responsibility of your health, making informed decisions, and being committed to lifelong healthier habits. That is what this book is all about - teaching you to take responsibility for your health and guiding you through that process.

There is a plethora of information on the Internet about how to prevent and 'cure' cancer. The challenge is making sense of it all and knowing where to begin. That's where The 7 Essentials steps come in.

---

1 http://www.cnn.com/2014/02/04/health/who-world-cancer-report/

2 http://stm.sciencemag.org/

3 http://www.ncbi.nlm.nih.gov/pmc/articles/PMC2515569/

This book will guide you through 7 key issues that will help ensure that you not only prevent Breast Cancer but also improve your odds of healing Breast Cancer.

TYPES OF BREAST CANCERS

What exactly is cancer? According to the National Cancer Institute, "Cancer is a term used for diseases in which abnormal cells divide without control and are able to invade other tissues. Cancer is just not one disease, but many diseases."[4]

There are basically 5 different types of Breast Cancer. The typical classifications used by medical doctors provide information about how the tumor grows and what kind of treatment they will prescribe.

HORMONE RECEPTOR, ESTROGEN, OR PROGESTERONE POSITIVE

The majority of Breast Cancers are estrogen positive (ER positive) or progesterone positive (PR positive). The ER positive cancers grow in response to the hormone estrogen while the PR positive cancers grow in response to progesterone. With the onslaught of environmental chemicals as well as all the chemicals found in personal care products that mimic estrogen, it comes as no big surprise that the majority of Breast Cancers are hormone receptor positive. Many of these false estrogens, also known as 'xeno-estrogens', can imitate estrogen and its effect on the body. These chemical estrogens are potent and powerful and have been found in extremely high levels in Breast Cancer tumors. An excess of estrogen and progesterone may also come as a result of poor methylation pathways and liver dysfunction. If you are not properly metabolizing these hormones, they can accumulate in the body. Further discussion about the false estrogens will be found in Chapter 3, Essential #2: Reduce Your Toxic Exposure.

Hormonal therapies for hormone receptor positive Breast Cancers are recommended after surgery, chemotherapy, and/or radiation. Typically, drugs like Tamoxifen, which block estrogen receptors on Breast Cancer cells, are prescribed for a minimum of 5 years.

---

[4] http://www.cancer.gov/cancertopics/cancerlibrary/what-is-cancer

Unbeknownst to most women, these drugs are classified as carcinogens by the World Health Organization and the American Cancer Society.[5]

Side effects of these drugs can double and even quadruple the risk of endometrial cancer in a five-year period. Other side effects can include stomach cancer, colon cancer, blood clots, fatty liver, memory impairment, and reduced sex drive.

HER2 POSITIVE BREAST CANCER

With this type of Breast Cancer, too much of the protein called HER2/neu (Human Epidermal Growth Factor Receptor) is produced. The HER2 gene creates a protein that plays an important role in *normal cell growth* and development. As a result of a genetic mutation or alteration in this gene, it begins to produce an increased amount of the growth factor receptor protein. This causes cells to divide and multiply more rapidly than normal.

The question is what causes the genetic mutation or alteration and can that be prevented? In the relatively new field of Epigenetics and Nutrigenomics, it has been found that specific nutrients and phytochemicals affect our gene expression and can actually turn genes on or off. As you will read in Chapter 7, Essential #6 - Repair with Therapeutic Plants, you will discover that plant based nutrients like curcumin and EGCG from green tea inhibits HER2 Breast Cancer cells. That's great news!

Herceptin is typically prescribed with HER2 positive Breast Cancers. Side effects of the drug include severe heart damage and possible lung damage.

---

[5] http://www.cancer.org/cancer/cancercauses/othercarcinogens/generalinformationaboutcarcinogens/known-and-probable-human-carcinogens

TRIPLE NEGATIVE BREAST CANCER

Triple negative Breast Cancers are named such because they are neither estrogen or progesterone receptor positive and do not overexpress the HER2 gene protein. Sometimes, the triple negative Breast Cancers tend to be more aggressive with a poor prognosis. Standard medical treatment consists of surgery, chemotherapy, and radiation.

DCIS-DUCTAL CELL CARCINOMA IN SITU

According to the Journal of the National Cancer Institute, DCIS is a condition of abnormal but not cancer cells that are found in the milk ducts.[6] The typical DCIS has not spread to nearby tissues and is often referred to as a 'pre-cancer'. DCIS was rarely diagnosed before the 1980s. With the increased push for mammography, the incidence of DCIS now represents 25% of all Breast Cancers that are diagnosed. Specifically, the risk of dying from DCIS within five years is less than 1%.

Although DCIS is not a true cancer, many of the treatments leave women confused about why they're being treated like they have invasive Breast Cancer. Is it possible that the lumpectomy, radiotherapy, and use of Tamoxifen eventually do cause a more aggressive cancer to develop? (More on that later.)

LOBULAR CARCINOMA IN SITU

Often referred to as lobular neoplasia, it doesn't seem to be an invasive cancer. It grows in the mill-producing glands of the breast. Like DCIS, it is considered a 'non-cancer'.

INFLAMMATORY BREAST CANCER

Also known as IBC, it is a rare and very aggressive type of Breast Cancer that accounts for 1%-5 % of Breast Cancers. The breast often appears swollen and inflamed since the cancer is blocking the lymph vessels in the skin of the breast. Since there is no 'lump', it cannot be

---

[6] http://www.cancer.gov/search/results

diagnosed with a mammogram. IBC is generally hormone receptor negative.

YOUR DNA IS NOT YOUR DESTINY

You have a great measure of control on the expression of your genes. The relatively new sciences of Epigenetics and Nutrigenomics have given us solid evidence that gene expressions can be changed. The old gene theory led us to believe that our genes and our DNA would ultimately express the outcome of our health and that we had very little control over it. How often have we heard the expression, "I inherited this from my mother or from my father"? Rather than being victims to our gene pool inheritance, we have the power to change and influence our genes in many ways.

According to Dr. Bruce Lipton, a world renowned cellular biologist and researcher in the field of quantum physics, the environment and not DNA shapes the development of our health. "Cellular biologists now recognized that the environment - the external universe and our internal physiology - and, more importantly, our perception of the environment directly control the activity of our genes." (The Biology of Belief: Unleashing the Power of Consciousness, Hay House 2008.)

There are many different types of signals that have an impact on our gene expression. Various influences such as your lifestyle choices, exposures to environmental toxins, dietary habits, and even our thoughts and feelings, can affect our gene expression.

A landmark study published by Dr. Dean Ornish M.D., clinical professor of medicine at the University of California, San Francisco, demonstrated that lifestyle changes could alter our genes.[7] Their study showed that improved nutrition, moderate exercise, stress management, and increased social support, changed the expression of over 500 genes. **These changes 'turned on' health-promoting genes while they 'turned off' genes that promoted heart disease, cancer, inflammation, and oxidative stress.**

---

[7] http://www.ornishspectrum.com/proven-program/the-research/

Genes can be turned off and on with the use of nutrition and specific antioxidants. For example, NRF2 is a gene that increases the cell antioxidant levels of glutathione. It can be activated and turned on with nutrients from broccoli sprouts and curcumin. Studies have shown and proven that your emotional and psychological state can also have an impact on your genes in your DNA.

A study conducted at the Institute of Heart Math, "Local and Nonlocal Effects of Fear," demonstrated the impact our emotions have on influencing our DNA.[8] Twenty-eight researchers were each given a vial containing DNA. They were instructed to feel positive feelings such as gratitude, love, and appreciation and project those feelings towards the DNA vial. In response to those emotions, the DNA relaxed, unwound, and lengthened.

Conversely, when the researchers emitted emotions such as stress, anger, and fear the DNA structure tightened, shortened, and switched off some of the gene codes. When they reverted back to normal, loving feelings, the DNA once again responded in a positive way.

In the Silva Mind Body Healing course[9], Laura Silva discusses a very similar experiment that was conducted by the military. The difference was that the DNA vials were in a separate room. While the subject was presented with different video clips that would stimulate various emotions, the emotional peaks and valleys of the test subject matched exactly the peaks and valleys in the reaction of the DNA. There was no lag time and no transmission time. The reaction was immediate.

They took the experiment one step further and carried the DNA vials over 50 miles away. Again, there was no lag time and no transmission time with the reaction of the donor.

In Chapter 5, Essential #5 – Heal Your Emotional Wounds, you'll come to understand how powerful your thoughts and emotions can be on the outcome of your health.

---

[8] http://appreciativeinquiry.case.edu/practice/organizationDetail.cfm?coid=852&sector=32

[9] http://mindvalley.directtrack.com/z/119/CD140/

7 CANCER TRIGGERS

In order to help you better understand how to be proactive with prevention and perhaps even heal your body, I have outlined seven major triggers that create cancer in the body. Remember that cancer is simply a symptom and not the cause.

Cancer cannot grow in a healthy body.

I will be reminding you of that several times throughout this book since it can be easy to fall back on the notion that this cancer 'just happened to me'. Remind yourself daily that your body has an amazing ability to heal and repair, given the proper nutrients, support, and proper lifestyle changes.

Since Breast Cancer is not one disease but a combination of many factors, it's important to take a step back and look at various triggers that may stimulate the growth of cancer in the body. Each of these topics will be discussed in more detail in each of The 7 Essentials.

TRIGGER #1- S.A.D. FOOD

The Standard America Diet's acronym (S.A.D.) is so appropriate. Processed, packaged and poisoned foods make up 90% of the grocery store shelves.

It is truly a sad state of affairs when traditional doctors don't know the difference between toxic food and healthy food. Here are a few of the main foods that trigger the growth of cancer cells.

EXCESSIVE SUGAR CONSUMPTION

Americans consume an average of 52 teaspoons of sugar per day![10] What most people don't realize is that cancer cells LOVE sugar. A study published in the International Journal of Endocrinology states: **"Cancer cells are well known to display an enhanced sugar uptake and consumption.** In fact, sugar transporters are deregulated in cancer cells so they incorporate higher amounts of sugar than normal cells."

---

[10] http://www.usda.gov/factbook/chapter2.pdf

It drives me crazy when I hear oncologists and medical physicians saying that there is no connection with sugar consumption and cancer. Visit any hospital or chemotherapy suite and you will see gobs of candy and sodas being offered to sick cancer patients.

The very technology that traditional medicine uses to detect cancer in various parts on the body is based on the premise that cancer LOVES sugar. A PET scan (Positron Emission Tomography) takes advantage of the cancer cells' voracious appetite for sugar and helps to determine the extent of the cancer in the body.

Before a PET scan, the patient is injected with a radioactive sugar solution. Since cancer has 10 times more insulin receptor sites compared to healthy cells, the cancer cells gobble up the radioactive sugar solution first. The end result is an image with little lights glowing in areas of the body that are afflicted with cancer cells.

There have been many books devoted to the effect of sugar on the human body. Suffice it to say, that since sugar comes in all shapes and forms, read your labels and avoid it like the plague. Limit your intake of carbs and whole grains as they eventually are broken down into simple sugars.

BAD FATS AND OILS

Fried foods served at fast food chains and restaurants, as well as many packaged and processed foods, contain hydrogenated oils that have been chemically altered. This allows for longer shelf and storage life. Aside from raising the 'bad cholesterol' (LDL) and lowering the 'good cholesterol' (HDL), these unhealthy oils damage the cell membrane. According to a renowned bio-chemist and cancer specialist, Dr. Johan Budwig, these dead oils "get into the cell membrane and destroy the electric charge of the membrane." When the electric charge is lost, the cells begin to suffocate because of lack of oxygen and turn to fermentation to survive; thus, the development of cancer.

ADDITIVES AND CHEMICALS

There are over 10,000 chemicals used in the food industry, most of which have never been tested for safety. Most food products that are manufactured and come out of a box are loaded with toxic chemicals. Many of the artificial colorings, flavorings, and additives have been linked to cancer and other auto immune diseases.[11]

HORMONES AND ANTIBIOTICS

There are six different kinds of steroid hormones[12] that are currently approved by the FDA for use in food production in the United States: estradiol, progesterone, testosterone, zeranol, trenbolone acetate, and melengestrol acetate. These hormones are used to increase the growth rate of cattle, sheep, and chickens. The hormone bGH is injected into cows to increase milk production. The large udders are continuously pumped which often leads to infections which results in the abuse of antibiotics.[13] The chronic exposure of the antibiotics to consumers from the dairy products has been linked to serious health risks such as drug resistant infections.

OVERCOOKED AND PROCESSED FOODS

Love potato chips and French fries? How about roasted breakfast cereals and certain snacks? Roasted coffee beans? Even the organic kind? If you do, read on.

The HEATOX project (Heat Generated Food Toxicants[14]) is a multi-disciplinary research project involving 14 countries. Knowing that hazardous by-products are produced when plant-based foods are cooked at high temperatures, (250° degrees Fahrenheit and above), HEATOX undertook studies of the effects of the various chemicals on the body. They identified more than 800 compounds that were produced as a result of heating foods at high temperatures, 52 of which are potential carcinogens.

---

[11] http://www.cspinet.org/reports/chemcuisine.htm
[12] http://envirocancer.cornell.edu/Factsheet/Diet/fs37.hormones.cfm
[13] http://www.pbs.org/wgbh/pages/frontline/shows/meat/safe/overview.html
[14] http://www.slv.se/upload/heatox/documents/D62_final_project_leaflet.pdf

One of the chemicals which especially caught their attention is called acrylamide. Acrylamide is so toxic and carcinogenic that the EPA has set a maximum contaminant level goal (MCLG) at 0 but has an allowable threshold of 0.2 micrograms per day.

So how much acrylamide are you getting when you eat your favorite potato chips? A report by the Environmental Law Foundation found that some potato chips had levels as high as 910 times the allowable threshold.[15]

According to their analysis, all the potato chip products tested required a 'warning' about the cancer risk because of the high levels of this cancer causing chemical.

The assessments of acrylamide in the HEATOX project are quite significant:

- There was an association with acrylamide levels and Breast Cancer
- Acrylamide, even at low doses, caused neurotoxicity in the fetus
- Acrylamide caused tumors in the intestines

TRIGGER #2 – ENVIRONMENTAL TOXICITY

Environmental toxicity includes all the chemicals we are exposed to in the environments, in our homes, and in our bodies. Let's look at the chemical chain from a macro level in the environment all the way down to the micro level inside your body.

The Environmental Working Group has created a beautiful but 'reality-shaking' video called 'The 10 Americans'.[16] The video poignantly demonstrates how deeply our toxic and polluted environment affects even an unborn child. In this study, a sample of blood from the cord of newborns was taken and tested for hundreds of chemical toxins. An average of 287 chemicals was found!

---

15 http://www.envirolaw.org/report_how_potato_chips_stack_up.pdf
16 http://www.ewg.org/news/videos/10-americans

Herbicides, pesticides, insecticides as well as many industrial compounds, fall into the category of 'Xeno-estrogens'. These chemicals mimic estrogens in the body and have been implicated in a variety of serious health problems, including cancer.

Let's take a closer look and see what toxicity lurks inside your home. Chemicals from carpeting, furniture, cleaning solutions, artificial air fresheners, scented candles, and even your pots and pans are contributing to a toxic environment.

Have you ever considered what you put ON your body? Your skin absorbs everything directly into the bloodstream. When you shower, brush your teeth, and pat yourself with all those potions and lotions, you are ingesting dangerous and toxic chemicals.

In fact, the average consumer is exposed to 127 chemicals per day, simply from their body care products.

Here are the chemicals found in a typical daily moisturizer.[17] Many of them are carcinogenic.

- Dimethicone (silica)
- PEG-50 Almond Glycerides
- Sodium Laureth Sulphate
- Cocoamidopropyl
- Triethanolamine (TEA)
- Methylchloroisothiazolinone
- Methyl Paraben
- FD&C Yellow No.6
- Fragrance

Lastly, when we think about toxicity, we must also look at the internal environment or terrain of the body. What is going on INSIDE the body that may be releasing toxins? Are you infected with parasites, bacteria, yeasts, fungi, and viruses?

---

[17] http://www.miessence.com/miessenceStory/ingredientsWeShun?lang=en&here=miessenceStory/ingredientsWeShun

Recent data from the Lancet Infectious Disease revealed that four types of chronic infections are associated with the development of cancer: HPV, H. pylori, Hepatitis B and C and Epstein Barr.[18]

There is another type of toxin that needs to be addressed, although it is not chemical in nature. We cannot see it, feel it, or taste it, but it affects us 24-7. It has become a hot topic of debate among scientists for the last decade. That toxin is called Electro-pollution.

Electro-pollution has been labeled the deadliest toxin on this planet. A wonderful objective study involving scientists from all over the world is called The Bio-Initiative Report.[19] ***The Bio-Initiative Report is an internationally acclaimed scientific and public health report on potential health risks of electromagnetic fields and radiofrequency/microwave radiation.***

According to the report: "Chronic exposure to EMF is associated with increased health risks that vary from impaired learning, headaches, mental confusion, skin rashes, tinnitus, and disorientation to a variety of cancers and neurological diseases like ALS and Alzheimer's. Sources of concern may include, but are not limited to, power lines, cell and cordless phones, cell towers, WI-FI, WIMax, and wireless internet."[20]

That pretty much sums up the world that we live in! There is no escaping it.

Dr. Devra Davis, a scientist, author, and professor, has done considerable research on the effects of cell phone radiation. She was appointed by several presidents, sat on a panel that was awarded a Nobel Prize, and she currently lectures at Harvard.

The title of her recent book tells it all: *Dissconnect. The Truth About Cell Phone Radiation, What The Industry Has Done To Hide it, And How To Protect Your Family.*[21]

---

18 http://www.cancer.med.umich.edu/news/virus.shtml

19 http://bioinitiative.org/freeaccess/index.htm

20 http://bioinitiative.org/freeaccess/editors/what.htm

21 http://astore.amazon.com/breacancconq-20?node=2&page=3

Here are a few facts:

- Cell phone radiation produces free radicals that weaken the DNA.
- Cell phone radiation weakens cell membranes.
- Cell phone radiation weakens the blood brain barrier.
- Children absorb more radiation than adults because their skulls are softer and their brains have more fluid.
- Sperm exposed to cell phone radiation die 4 times faster and are biologically damaged.
- Keeping an iPhone 4 in your pocket exceeds the FCC exposure guidelines. (It's in the fine print warnings that come with your cell phone.)
- A 2008 study that Dr. Davis sites in her book concluded that the radio-frequency from 3G phones caused 10 times more DNA damage than the 2G phones. So what kind of damage are 4G phones doing?
- Many physicians have seen a correlation with Breast Cancers and tumors and women who *use their bra as a holding device for their cell phone*.

Cell phones release constant doses of non-ionizing radiation that increases free radical production and causes DNA damage.

If you store your cell phone in your bra or keep it close to your body all day long, you are dousing your sensitive breast tissue with radiation.

In the May 2012 issue of the *Environmental Health Trust Newsletter*[22], cancer specialists discuss the unusual case of multiple breast tumors on a young woman who used her bra as a cell phone carrier. The doctors could actually trace the shape of her cell phone by the number of small multiple tumors she had!

Another area of the body that is particularly sensitive to non-ionizing cell phone radiation are the hormonal glands. According to Dr.

---

[22] http://ehtrust.org/books-publications/newsletters/

Andrew Goldsworthy from the Imperial College in London, glandular cells are particularly sensitive to radiation. "Although electromagnetic fields frequently stimulate glandular activity in the short term, long-term exposure is often harmful in that the gland ceases to work properly."[23]

Of particular interest is the Thyroid Gland and the Breast Cancer connection.

When you hold your cell phone near your head, you are exposing your thyroid gland to non-ionizing radiation. If you are sitting in front of a computer for several hours per day, you are exposing your thyroid to another source of EMF.

Studies have shown that after three months exposure to power-line frequencies, the thyroid glands of rats showed visible signs of deterioration. They also lost their ability to produce the thyroid hormones, which they did not recover from, even after the fields were switched off. Similar visible deterioration of the thyroid gland was found in rats exposed to simulated 2G cell phone radiation for 20 minutes a day for three weeks.

People living for six years within 100 meters of a cell phone base station have shown a significant reduction in the release into the blood of a number of hormones, including ACTH from the pituitary gland, cortisol from the adrenal glands, and testosterone. However, the most highly significant loss was in their ability to produce the thyroid hormones. The expected consequence of this is hypothyroidism.[24]

According to an article in Breast Cancer Research, scientists have noted an increased prevalence of thyroid disease in patients with Breast Cancer.[25]

At first sight, this information may seem overwhelming and that there is no escaping the EMF's that are looming around us 24/7. After all,

---

[23] http://stopsmartmeters.org.uk/wp-content/uploads/2012/04/Biol-Effects-EMFs-2012-NZ1.pdf

[24] http://stopsmartmeters.org.uk/wp-content/uploads/2012/04/Biol-Effects-EMFs-2012-NZ1.pdf

[25] http://www.ncbi.nlm.nih.gov/pmc/articles/PMC314438/

we can't live in a bubble, and we all choose to live with our electronic devices. So what is the solution? There have been huge advancements in scientifically valid technology that neutralizes the effects of the EMF's on our bodies.[26] The details of that will be discussed in Chapter 3, Essential #2: Reduce Your Toxic Exposure.

TRIGGER #3 – PHYSICAL AND HORMONAL STRESS

According to Dr. Carl Rubia, Nobel Prize Laureate, our physical body is comprised of only 1 billionth physical matter...the rest is all energy. Since we are energetic beings, it is vital to keep our energy flowing, so to speak.

Our cells communicate with each other through photon light. Our nerve system commands and controls every function in the body through electrical pathways and our organs communicate with each other through the acupuncture meridian system. With all this energetic exchange going on, it is so important to make sure that there is no obstruction in that energy flow. Obstructions can occur because of spinal subluxations, chemical toxicities, and chronic emotional stress.

Another form of stress that occurs in our body is called Oxidative Stress. Oxidative Stress is the body's inability to readily detoxify or repair damage from toxins.[27] When your body breaks down food, or when it is exposed to environmental toxins, it produces free radicals which can cause DNA and cellular damage. If your liver and detoxification pathways are not functioning at optimal levels, the chronic exposure of the free radicals can lead to DNA damage and ultimately cancer.

Hormonal stress affects us in many ways. Women especially can attest to the fact that when their hormones are out of balance, they FEEL out of balance. Since estrogen is intricately involved with so many hormonal pathways, the concern about these foreign estrogens is that they are interfering with reproduction, increasing endometriosis, increasing fibroids in the uterus and breasts, affecting sperm

---

[26] http://giawellness.com/drveronique/products/terra-gia/

[27] http://en.wikipedia.org/wiki/Oxidative_stress

production, and increasing the possibility of developing Breast Cancer.

A study posted in an article in the *Journal of Applied Toxicology* revealed high concentrations of parabens in post-mastectomy breasts affected with Breast Cancer.[28] The parabens were present even with women who had never used any type of underarm deodorant throughout their whole lifetime, indicating that the parabens were acquired through the cosmetic, food, and pharmaceutical industries.

If you cannot metabolize or properly breakdown all of these foreign estrogens, you get a buildup of the more 'aggressive' proliferative estrogen.

Imbalanced estrogen can trigger abnormal cells to divide and has been associated with many female cancers such as breast, uterine, and ovarian.

TRIGGER #4 – EMOTIONAL WOUNDS

Although the complex relationship between 'psychology and physiology' is not clearly understood, scientists are well aware that psychological stress affects the immune system.

C.W. Douglas Brodie, MD[29], a physician who was an early pioneer in Alternative Medicine, worked with cancer patients for over 28 years. He found specific traits that showed up over and over in the thousands of cancer patients with which he worked. Here are the 7 basic traits that he felt induced emotional stress that was a causative factor in developing cancer:

- Being highly conscientious, caring, dutiful, responsible, and hard-working.
- Someone who 'worries for others' and carries other people's burdens.
- A 'people pleaser' with a great need for approval.

---

[28] http://www.ncbi.nlm.nih.gov/pubmed/14745841
[29] http://www.cancure.org/dr_brodie.htm

- Poor relationship with one or both parents and usually the spouse.
- Internalizes toxic emotions like anger and resentment and has great difficulty expressing these emotions.
- Unable to cope adequately with stress.
- Has unresolved deep-seated emotional problems and conflicts from childhood and are often unaware of their presence.

Dr. R.G. Hamer[30], a renowned German physician and cancer surgeon, examined over 20,000 patients with all types of cancer. By comparing x-rays of their brains and the location of the cancer in the body, Dr. Hamer came to this conclusion:

***"I searched for cancer in the cell,
and I have found it in the brain."***

Dr. Hamer felt that any cancer began with an extremely harsh emotional shock that would 'short circuit' a specific area of the brain and then would, in turn, weaken a particular organ and make it more vulnerable to cancer.

TRIGGER #5 – DENTAL TOXICITIES

I have personally consulted with thousands of patients with compromised Immune Systems over the years and found that they had a common denominator - dental toxicities. Dental toxicities affect you in 2 ways: chemically and energetically.

'Silver' fillings are a hodge - podge of metals including mercury, nickel, cadmium, silver, and copper. Mercury is the most toxic, naturally occurring substance on the planet. There is NO SAFE level of mercury; yet, there are many naysayers including dentists, doctors, and patients who refuse to accept these facts.

Chronic mercury poison can directly and indirectly contribute to and increase the risk and severity of every known disease and health issue.

---

[30] http://learninggnm.com/documents/hamerbio.html

In a 5 year study with Breast Cancer patients, Dr. Robert Jones found that 93% of women he worked with had root canals.[31] He also found that the tumors were, in the majority of the cases, on the same side as the root canal.

The internationally recognized medical researcher, Yoshiaki Omura, M.D., has studied the effects of heavy metals on the body, and he believes all cancer cells have mercury in them.[32]

Metal fillings, root canals, and metal implants act as virtual antenna and can attract and make you more susceptible to the effects of Electro-Pollution.[33]

According to Lina Garcia, DDS, DMD, who is associated with Dr. Mercola's Natural Health Care Center in Chicago:[34]

"When considering the numerous reasons for the increasing prevalence of chronic illness in our society, I think that we should not overlook the possibility that metal-containing dental work, especially titanium implants, could be acting like antennas for the microwave transmissions going on between our cell phones and all of the cell phone towers in our 21st century environment. I strongly suspect that this is an unrecognized source of insidious stress on our physical, mental, and emotional health."[35]

TRIGGER #6 – INFLAMMATION AND METHYLATION

This section may be a little technical, but it is an important aspect to understand. Don't worry if you don't 'get it' at first. It took me a while to put it all together. I happened to stumble across this after I had

---

[31] http://articles.mercola.com/sites/articles/archive/2012/02/18/dangers-of-root-canaled-teeth.aspx

[32] http://imva.info/index.php/2010/05/heavy-metals-mercury-and-cancer/

[33] http://articles.mercola.com/sites/articles/archive/2012/08/25/heavy-metal-electromagnetic-fields.aspx#_edn2

[34] http://mercuryfreedentists.com/mercury-free-dentists/illinois/dr.-lina-garcia-dds.-dmd.html

[35] http://articles.mercola.com/sites/articles/archive/2012/08/25/heavy-metal-electromagnetic-fields.aspx#_edn2

some blood work done and my Homocysteine levels were off the charts! I was a stroke and heart attack waiting to happen!

How and why was my Homocysteine so high since I had an excellent diet, had a regular supplementation regime, and exercised regularly?

This brought me down the road of research and discovery. Although this trigger is closely related to diet and lifestyle, I felt it was important to put it into its own separate category. The effects of inflammation and methylation can be improved with healthier eating habits and proper supplementation.

The role of inflammation and Breast Cancer has become abundantly clear. It has been estimated that 95% of all cancers have a common factor:

Inflammation and a protein complex involved in cellular stress called NF-kB.

"Interestingly, inflammation[36] functions at all 3 stages of tumor development: initiation, progression, and metastasis. Inflammation contributes to initiation. Chronic inflammation appears to contribute to tumor progression by establishing a milieu conducive to the development of different cancers."

In a study funded by the National Institutes of Health, the Cancer Research Journal reported that the inflammatory process in the breast can promote cancer stem cells responsible for developing Breast Cancer. On the flip side, scientists were also able to demonstrate that inactivating the inflammatory factor NF-kB resulted in reduced activity of Breast Cancer stem cells and prevented the cancer from forming.

The inflammatory trigger is a very powerful piece of the puzzle for healing and preventing Breast Cancer.

What causes inflammation that may increase your risk for Breast Cancer?

---

[36] http://cancerres.aacrjournals.org/content/65/19/8583.full

- Smoking and Alcohol.
- Sleep deficit.
- Environmental toxins, both in and out of the home.
- Unhealthy saturated fats, trans fats, and too many Omega 6's.
- Chronic elevated blood sugar and insulin resistance.
- Chronic stress.

Methylation is a complex bio-chemical process that occurs in our bodies every day. Think of methylation like the spark plug in a car that evokes certain chemical reactions. Methylation causes hormones and proteins to 'change' into different substances. For example, methylation helps convert serotonin into melatonin. It helps change 'strong' estrogens to milder, less aggressive estrogens.

Methylation is also crucial for the proper expression of DNA and detoxification pathways. Scientists have shown that cancer cells have abnormal methylation. When methylation does not occur, unhealthy genes get turned on and healthy genes get turned off.

Studies specifically about Breast Cancer and methylation issues are uncovering another important piece of the puzzle. Scientists are finding that improper methylation patterns:

- Lead to inactivation of certain genes in the breast tissue.[37]
- Is commonly associated with Breast Cancer.
- Breast Cancer prognosis is closely linked to methylation[38]
- Methylation plays an important role in the development of certain types of Breast Cancer.[39]

How do you know if you have methylation problems? There are simple urine tests[40] that can be done in the privacy of your home and then sent to a laboratory to be analyzed. DNA Genomic testing is also a simple way to discover your methylation pathways.

---

[37] http://www.ncbi.nlm.nih.gov/pubmed/17090521
[38] http://www.ncbi.nlm.nih.gov/pubmed/2068666
[39] http://www.ncbi.nlm.nih.gov/pubmed/20565864
[40] http://breastcancerconqueror.com/store/products/category/hormone-testing/

In Chapter 7, you will learn how to repair inflammation and poor methylation with the use of specific herbs and supplements.

TRIGGER #7 – NEEDLES & KNIVES, LOTIONS & POTIONS

This last trigger is what is known as iatrogenic or medically induced cancers. What may come as a shock to many, the very instruments that are used to diagnose and treat cancer, are some of the very causes of cancer.

The *July 2013 issue of JAMA*[41] clearly confirms that over-diagnosis leads to over treatment which can be potentially harmful. Women undergoing traditional breast screenings with mammograms have over a 50% chance of being diagnosed with a 'false positive'. That means that if they find a benign tumor like DCIS, the patient may be encouraged to have biopsies, surgery, radiation, and sometimes even chemotherapy for a cyst that has not developed into cancer....yet. But with the barrage of assaults to the breast, it often does develop into cancer.[42]

According to Medscape News, "The practice of oncology is in need of a host of reforms."[43] It is a well-known scientific fact that stem cells that are subjected to needless radiation and chemical poisoning actually stimulate the growth of the cancer and make it more malignant.[44]

According to Dr. Allen Levin, M.D., author of The Healing of Cancer,

> ***"The majority of the cancer patients in this country die because of chemotherapy, which does not cure breast, colon, or lung cancer. This has been documented for over a decade and nevertheless doctors still utilize chemotherapy to fight these tumors."***

Let's begin with the use of medical radiation.

---

[41] http://jama.jamanetwork.com/article.aspx?articleid=1722196

[42] http://breastcancerconqueror.com/treatments-for-dcis-cause-cancer/

[43] http://www.medscape.com/viewarticle/808654

[44] http://www.greenmedinfo.com/blog/chemo-and-radiation-actually-make-cancer-more-malignant

CT SCANS:

Research by the Radiation Epidemiology Branch of the National Cancer Institute suggests that CT scans in the US in 2007 may have produced 29,000 cancers, *about 6% of them being Breast Cancer.*[45]

DENTAL X-RAYS:

According to the Journal of the American Dental Association, "Dentists should NOT prescribe routine dental radiographs at preset intervals for all patients."[46] The radiation penetrates the brain and thyroid gland.

RADIATION 'THERAPY:

Exposure to ionizing radiation through 'radiation therapy' has clearly been established as one of the risk factors for the development of Breast Cancer.[47] Increased risk is associated with increased exposures.

Researchers from the Department of Radiation Oncology at the UCLA Jonsson Comprehensive Cancer Center report that ***radiation treatment actually drives Breast Cancer cells into greater malignancy***. They found that even when radiation kills half of the tumor cells treated, the surviving cells which are resistant to treatment, known as induced Breast Cancer stem cells (iBCSCs), were up to 30 times more likely to form tumors than the non-irradiated Breast Cancer cells.[48]

MAMMOGRAMS:

I am not a fan of mammography because of the many serious side effects of radiation and compression of the breast. A meta-analysis of

---

[45] http://dceg.cancer.gov/about/organization/programs-ebp/reb

[46] http://jada.ada.org/content/137/9/1304.full?sid=0915e473-6fd9-400a-a813-619938091556

[47] http://www.ncbi.nlm.nih.gov/pubmed/19930978

[48] http://www.greenmedinfo.com/blog/study-radiation-therapy-can-make-cancers-30x-more-malignant

127 studies concluded that low dose radiation increases Breast Cancer risk among high-risk women.[49]

Cancer research in the UK suggests that a decade of annual two-view mammographic screening before age 40 years would result in a net increase in Breast Cancer deaths.[50]

Although DCIS is not considered a 'true cancer', it is unfortunately treated as such. Most doctors recommend a lumpectomy and radiation 'therapy'. Sadly, the radiation often results in the likelihood of a mastectomy.[51] (More than likely the radiation caused real cancer to develop and the innocent women think they have no choice but to have their breast cut off.)

According to Dr. Samuel Epstein, an international leading authority on the causes and prevention of cancer, 2 X-ray films of a breast in premenopausal woman gives about 500 times the dose of a chest x ray.[52]

Extend that over a 10 year period and the accumulated radiation is close to the kind of dosage that women got in Hiroshima outside the major epicenter where the atom bomb exploded.

UNNECESSARY SURGERY

There are times when surgery can be a lifesaving procedure and necessary to save the life of a patient. On the other hand, we have all heard the horrifying stories of cancer patients undergoing surgery to remove a simple tumor and months later the cancer has spread all over their body. Doctors are very well aware that surgery causes the cancer to spread and it also suppresses the Immune System.[53] *The British Journal of Cancer* agreed by stating, ***"The primary tumor***

---

[49] http://www.ncbi.nlm.nih.gov/pubmed/20582702

[50] http://www.ncbi.nlm.nih.gov/pubmed/16136033

[51] http://www.ncbi.nlm.nih.gov/pubmed/21720992

[52] http://www.preventcancer.com/publications/pdf/Interview%20%20June%2003.htm

[53] http://journals.lww.com/annalsofsurgery/Abstract/2011/04000/Improving_Postoperative_Immune_Status_and.24.aspx

***removal may result in sudden acceleration of the metastatic process."*[54]**

Here are some earth shattering facts in response to surgical removal of a tumor.

- During the surgical procedure, natural barriers that contain the tumor are breached, enabling cancer cells to escape their original confinement and spread to other parts of the body.
- Surgery induces immune suppression while initiating an inflammatory cascade that provides cancer cells to propagate.
- In response to the trauma, the body secretes growth factors to facilitate the healing. Unfortunately, these same growth factors also stimulate tumor cell growth.
- Cancer spill into the blood stream from the surgical margins and establish metastatic colonies in other parts of the body.
- Cancer cells have a 'Velcro like' surface that allows them to stick to each other and the blood vessel walls. In one experiment that mimicked surgical conditions, the sticking and binding of cancer cells to blood vessel walls increased by 250%.
- Surgery reduces the Natural Killer Cell activity. NK cells' function is to gobble up cancer cells.

Do needle biopsies fall into that same category? Absolutely! ***Manipulation of an intact tumor with needle biopsies is associated with an increased risk of metastasis or spread of the cancer.*[55]**

The tumor is encased with a thick wall, but once a needle is inserted into the protective wall, fluid containing millions of cancer cells can escape into the blood and lymphatic system. Often times the biopsy is repeated several times, increasing the risk for spreading. A titanium 'marker' is often inserted into the breast tissue in order to make the area more easily visible on x-rays and sonograms. Titanium is a toxic

---

[54] http://www.nature.com/bjc/index.html

[55] http://archsurg.jamanetwork.com/article.aspx?articleid=396893

metal and I have repeatedly seen unsuspecting women react with inflammation and pain as a result of the titanium implant.

It's YOUR body. Ask questions!

When I have blogged about similar information, women write to me, explaining that it was important for them to know what cancer they had, simply for their peace of mind. They wanted to know what they were dealing with. I understand that completely. The decision is yours to make. Weigh the risk of the cancer possibly spreading versus the benefits of having a label to the cancer.

There are less traumatic ways of discovering how much cancer you are actually producing with simple blood tests that are very sensitive markers. One of these tests is the TK1 test which measures the activity of the TK1 enzymes that are produced when cancer cells are dividing.[56] This diagnostic tool has been around for 30 years and has been used in over 30 countries. There are hundreds of peer review studies that have verified the accuracy of this simple test. You can read more about this test in Chapter 8: Adopt Very Early Detection.

TOXIC DRUGS AND CHEMICALS

I once had a patient who described her AHA moment to me about her chemotherapy experience. In her words, "I was sitting in this room full of women that looked like death. I was waiting for my turn to have my weekly dose of chemo inserted through my port. As I watched the nurse handle the bag of fluid with gloves and a mask, I noticed that the bag had this big 'CAUTION' sign on it. ***It dawned on me that if it was too toxic for her to handle without gloves, why was I feeding that poison into my body?*** I got up, politely said, "No Thank You," walked out, and never looked back."

The history of chemotherapy drugs can be traced to chemical warfare during World War 1.[57] After a German Air raid in Bari, Italy, more than 1000 people were exposed to the chemical warfare agent 'nitrogen mustard'. Autopsies of the victims were examined by an

---

[56] http://breastcancerconqueror.com/stop-breast-cancer-before-it-starts/

[57] http://en.wikipedia.org/wiki/History_of_cancer_chemotherapy

expert in chemical warfare. He found that there was profound suppression of lymphoid and myeloid tissue as a result of the exposure to the mustard gas.

In his 'not so divine' wisdom, he surmised that this chemical could then be used against cancer cells in order to stop their rapid division. Thus, began the era of toxic chemotherapies.

When you take a step back, and look at the facts in a logical way, does it really make sense to insert a poison in a body that is already compromised and weak? The dismal statistics of chemotherapeutic agents speak for themselves.

The Department of Radiation Oncology in Sydney Australia undertook a study involving 22 major adult cancers and relationship to the benefits of the use of chemotherapy treatments alone.58 Their conclusion:

"The overall contribution of curative and adjuvant cytotoxic chemotherapy to 5-year survival in adults was estimated to be 2.3% in Australia and 2.1% in the USA."

In other words, with the use of chemotherapy alone, you have a 2% chance of surviving your cancer.

Other drugs that are used to 'treat' Breast Cancer include estrogen blockers such as Tamoxifen and hormone blocking drugs (aromatase inhibitors) such as Arimidex, Aromasin, and Femara.

Tamoxifen is an antagonist of estrogen receptors,59 which means it blocks the estrogen receptor on the Breast Cancer cell. Think of an estrogen receptor on a cell like a key hole and the estrogen fits perfectly into that key hole. Tamoxifen acts by binding with that 'key hole' on the cell and, thus, blocks out the estrogen.

In theory, that sounds like a positive action in estrogen driven Breast Cancers. But in reality, Tamoxifen has serious side effects, driving cancers into other areas of the body. In fact, Tamoxifen doubles and

---

[58] http://www.ncbi.nlm.nih.gov/pubmed/?term=contribution+of+cytotoxic+chemotherpay+to+5+year+survival+in+adult+malignancies

[59] http://en.wikipedia.org/wiki/Tamoxifen

even quadruples the risk of endometrial cancer in a five year period.60 Other side effects include: stomach cancer, colon cancer, blood clots, fatty liver, memory impairment, and a reduced sex drive.61

How does that make sense? Prescribe a cancer causing drug and cross your fingers and hope that it does not cause another type of cancer? I can't make any sense out of that logic.

Here are a few of the side effects of the Hormone Blocking Drugs:

- Use of Aromatase inhibitors is associated with Vitamin D deficiency.[62]
- Decreases estrogen for only 12 months but not 24 months.[63]
- Significantly increases levels of IGF-1, Insulin Growth Factor, which ***increases growth of cancer cells.***[64]
- Causes cognitive deficits (makes your brain sluggish).[65]
- Over 71% of women experience musculoskeletal complaints.[66]
- Contributes to decline of bone mineral density and increased fractures.[67]
- Functional impairment of hands because of tendon-synovial changes.[68]
- Increases in_hot flashes.[69]

Since conventional treatments offer such serious risks and stimulate cancer production I believe this is why so many women are looking for safer and gentler ways to heal their body. Women around the

---

[60] http://www.iss.it/publ/anna/2006/2/422170.pdf
[61] http://www.greenmedinfo.com/article/adjuvant-tamoxifen-therapy-early-stage-breast-cancer-increases-risk-second-primarly
[62] http://www.ncbi.nlm.nih.gov/pubmed/20399042
[63] http://www.ncbi.nlm.nih.gov/pubmed/19967558
[64] http://www.ncbi.nlm.nih.gov/pubmed/19967558
[65] http://www.ncbi.nlm.nih.gov/pubmed/20097718
[66] http://www.ncbi.nlm.nih.gov/pubmed/20035381
[67] http://www.ncbi.nlm.nih.gov/pubmed/20429308
[68] http://www.ncbi.nlm.nih.gov/pubmed/18474874
[69] http://www.ncbi.nlm.nih.gov/pubmed/16870085

globe that have communicated with me, all share the same desire: They want to be heard. They want to have a voice in their course of treatment. They want their doctors to work with them as they are on a healing journey with evidence based natural medicine. I pray that this book will be that for you: a guidebook and companion that will not only inform and educate but that will also encourage you to open your heart and mind to new possibilities of healing.

THE 'PINK' FRENZY

Unfortunately, Breast Cancer is associated with those darn pink ribbons. I don't know about you, but I get really frustrated with the pink ribbon movement. What has the pink ribbon done to reduce Breast Cancer rates? Nothing! What has it done to find 'the cure'? Nothing! Instead it lures women into a false sense of security with 'Breast Cancer Awareness' with more mammograms.

You may be surprised to learn that the original 'pink ribbon' was salmon colored, and it was designed to put the National Cancer Institute on notice about the lack of funding for the prevention of Breast Cancer. Charlotte Haley was trying to make a statement to the NCI after her mother, sister, and daughter had all been diagnosed with Breast Cancer. She came from her heart and was sincere about creating awareness about the prevention of Breast Cancer.

Estee Lauder loved Charlotte's idea of the ribbon and wanted to join forces with her to raise money for Breast Cancer, while promoting her toxic perfumes and skin products. Well, Charlotte quickly saw where that was headed and refused her offer. Estee Lauder stole the ribbon idea and changed the color to pink....and you know the rest of the story.

Fast forward to Breast Cancer Awareness Month. It should come as no surprise that the mega pharmaceutical company Astra Zeneca and Imperial Chemical Industry initiated this yearly campaign.

I think Dr. Samuel Epstein, a medical researcher of occupational and environmental medicine at the University of Illinois School of Public Health, said it best:[70]

"This is a conflict of interest unparalleled in the history of American medicine."

"You have got a company that's a spin-off of one of the world's biggest manufacturers of carcinogenic chemicals: they have control of Breast Cancer treatment, and they have got control of chemoprevention. They have got control over the public message of National Breast Cancer Awareness Month, which focuses on early detection and **not prevention.**"

The Breast Cancer Action[71] is the watchdog of the Breast Cancer Movement. Because they do not accept any funding from entities that profit from or contribute to cancer, they are able to speak the TRUTH about the Breast Cancer Industry. They have created a 'Think Before You Pink'[72] campaign that is designed to bring awareness about the growing concern of the pink ribbon products and promotions. They encourage you to ask critical questions about the Pink Ribbon Movement and the mass 'pinkwashing' that pharmaceutical companies and medical organizations promote.

My frustration with this pink ribbon movement helped me create my own personal icon for Breast Cancer. ***I chose the purple butterfly. (or should I say the purple butterfly chose me? ☺)***

Some of my best creative ideas come as a result of a meditation and quiet time. One sunny afternoon, I was feeling particularly impatient about my own healing journey. I kept asking questions. "Why am I going through this? Why is this taking so long to heal? What more can I do to facilitate my physical and emotional healing?"

Then clear as day, I saw this image in my mind of a cocoon being transformed into a beautiful butterfly. The short and stubby

[70] http://www.preventcancer.com/publications/pdf/Interview%20%20June%2003.htm

[71] http://thinkbeforeyoupink.org/?page_id=12

[72] http://thinkbeforeyoupink.org/

caterpillar goes through 3 stages of transformation and metamorphosis so that the beautiful butterfly can emerge. The cocoon 'surrenders' in full faith as it goes through this transition, knowing that this vulnerability will lead to full expression and expansion.

The butterfly has to be patient as it goes through its transformation, waiting until it has completely matured before it can emerge. Philosophers and naturalists have described the butterfly as the representation of freedom and liberty.

A Breast Cancer healing journey is very similar to that of a butterfly. You may start out having certain beliefs, habits, and lifestyles but if you open your heart and mind, and are patient, you will see that your Breast Cancer journey is more than just healing your body physically. It is also about transforming the inner you. You will come to understand that your healing journey has a greater purpose - that you will emerge on the 'other side' as a happier, healthier, more-fulfilled, and spiritual you.

Let's begin the journey together.....

POINTS TO PONDER

- More than half of all cancers are preventable.
- Your DNA is NOT your destiny. The science of Epigenetics has proven that what I choose to eat can positively impact my gene expression.
- Cancer cannot grow in a healthy body. The body has to be 'diseased', tired, and toxic in order for cancer to develop.
- There are 7 main Cancer Triggers that can be prevented.
- Eating a typical S.A.D. will result in the standard chronic illnesses.
- Environmental toxicity, macro and micro, are responsible for stressing the Immune System and detoxification pathways.
- There are many 'foreign estrogens' or Xeno-estrogens that can stimulate Breast Cancer.

- There is a strong connection between emotional trauma and the development of Breast Cancer.
- Dental toxins impact my health through bacterial and metal toxins as well as the blockage of energetic meridian flow.
- Inflammation and poor methylation are key factors in setting the stage for the development of Breast Cancer.
- Unfortunately, there are too many medically induced cancers.
- The Pink Ribbon campaign has done absolutely nothing to help prevent and cure Breast Cancer.

YOUR HEALING JOURNEY ACTION STEPS

1.) Write down everything you put in your mouth over the course of the next 3 days and simply make an observation about how it compares to the S.A.D. diet.

Breakfast

Lunch

Dinner

Snacks

2.) Make a list of household cleaners and anything 'artificial and chemical' that are in your home. Read the ingredients.

3.) Take a moment to notice how your body feels at various times during the day. Is your neck tight? Do you feel stressed? Do your hormones feel out of balance? Take a moment to jot down your thoughts.

4.) Notice how you feel about the majority of your relationships. Are they supportive or negative? Look back at the last 2 years and reflect on any major stressful event that may have occurred. Don't dwell on it, simply jot it down. We will get into some Emotional releasing and healing in a few more chapters.

5.) Take a few minutes to look inside your mouth and jot down the number of fillings, crowns, and root canals that you have.

6.) Make list of all the various over the counter and prescribed drugs that you take on a regular basis.

CHAPTER 2

ESSENTIAL #1 - LET FOOD BE YOUR MEDICINE

"If man made it, don't eat it."

~

Jack Lalane

STOP FEEDING THE CANCER

As previously discussed, the acronym for the Standard American Diet, SAD, is quite appropriate. The standard American diet has brought nothing but pain and disease to a country that claims to be at the forefront of so many technologies. According to a 2011 poll by *Consumer Reports Health*[73], 9:10 Americans believe they have a healthy diet, although 43% of them still drink at least 1 sugar filled soda every day. Forty percent of the people polled said they ate "pretty much everything that they wanted." According to the poll, Americans tend to give themselves high marks for 'healthy eating', although their definition of healthy eating consisted of sugary drinks, fatty foods, and few fruits and vegetables.

---

[73] http://news.discovery.com/human/health/americans-diet-weight-110104.htm

The science of studying the effect of nutrition in our everyday foods has taught us how incredibly powerful these life-sustaining nutrients can be.

According to an article in the *Nutrition Journal*, with a diet comprised of a proper balance of healthy oils, cruciferous vegetables, trace minerals, enzymes and probiotics, as well as specific supplements, it is likely that there could be at least a 60% to 70% decrease in the development of Breast Cancer.[74]

The World Health Organization contends that many common cancers, including Breast Cancer, may be influenced by such things as diet, environmental factors, and lifestyle choices. A study conducted by the University of Montréal found that women who consumed 27 different fruits and vegetables per week reduce the risk of Breast Cancer by an amazing 73%.[75]

So it all boils down to this: what you choose to eat is either feeding your body or feeding the cancer.

It really can be that simple. Let's take a look at a few key foods that must be avoided if you want to starve the cancer.

CANCER LOVES ACIDIC FOOD

The entire metabolic process of the human body depends on one critical factor - the pH of the plasma fluids. The pH scale is very simple. The lower the readings on the pH scale are acidic and the higher readings are more alkaline. Through homeostasis, the body maintains a healthy plasma pH of 7.4. Although the pH of the body will fluctuate with meals, exercise, stress, hormones, and sleep, a healthy and balanced first-morning saliva pH should be between 7.0 to 7.4.

A simple principle to apply concerning health and disease is that a low pH creates an environment conducive to dis-ease and a higher, alkaline pH promotes health.

---

[74] http://www.nutritionj.com/content/pdf/1475-2891-3-19.pdf

[75] http://www.anticancerbook.com/post/Genes-that-are-hungry-for-fruits-vegetables-and-fish.html

When the scales tip in favor of an acidic micro-environment, a domino effect is created. Toxins are not properly excreted which creates a favorable environment for pathogens such as bacteria, viruses, and yeasts to thrive. Also, prolonged irritation of the cell membrane from environmental carcinogens blocks the intake of much needed oxygen. When the cell lacks oxygen, it creates lactic acid and becomes acidic. This creates the perfect environment for cancer cells to develop and multiply.[76]

The very nature of cancer is that it flourishes in a very acidic environment.

The surrounding tissue that is found in cancer tumors has a very low pH, meaning that it is very acidic. In order to stop feeding the cancer, your focus is to avoid acidic foods and move towards alkaline foods.

ALKALINE FOODS:

- Vegetables
- Herbal Teas
- Certain fruits
- Vegetable broths
- Green drinks
- Unsweetened nut milks
- Vegetable juices
- Raw, soaked nuts
- Clean water with lemon
- Coconut, olive, flax, hemp oils
- Clean water with 1 tsp. baking soda
- Sprouted seeds

ACIDIC FOODS

- All meats except salmon

[76] http://www.ncbi.nlm.nih.gov/pubmed/22380870

- Dairy products
- What pastas and breads
- Sodas, beer, alcohol
- Most grains
- Vegetable oils, saturated fats
- Most condiments
- Salted, roasted nuts
- Sugar containing foods
- White vinegar
- Processed, packaged foods
- Microwaved meals

THE TOP 7 FOODS TO AVOID

SUGAR

If there is one food that has to be eliminated from your diet, it is sugar. There is no dancing around that one except facing the fact right away. Since cancer cells have twice the number of insulin receptor sites compared to a healthy cell, it would make sense that the first thing you would avoid like the plague would be sugar. It has been known since 1923 that tumor cells use a lot more glucose than normal cells. Knowing this fact alone can help you control tumor growth.

A study done at UCLA proved how simple it was to kill cancer cells: deprive them of glucose.[77] The researchers discovered that depriving cancer cells of glucose or sugar activated metabolic pathways that lead to cancer cell death.

Another way in which sugar affects the growth of cancer cells is by stimulating high insulin and insulin like growth factors. IGF-1 (insulin growth factors) can directly promote tumor cell growth by the insulin/IGF signaling pathway. Conversely, when blood sugar levels

---

[77] http://www.sciencedaily.com/releases/2012/06/120626131854.htm

are low and ketone bodies are elevated, this negatively impacts the proliferation of malignant cells.[78]

Sugar comes in all shapes and forms and sizes. Here is a basic list of sugars that must be avoided:

- White refined sugar
- Brown sugar
- Simple carbohydrates from grains turn to sugar very quickly. This would include all breads and pastas made from white flour.
- White rice
- Honey
- Agave
- Maple Syrup
- High fructose corn syrup is a major source of sugar in the North American diet, to the tune of 150 grams of sugar per day or 30 teaspoons per day!
- All fruits, except green apples, lemons and limes, and occasionally a few berries.
- Wine, beers and liquors
- All artificial sweeteners in the pink, blue, or yellow packets

Some of you may be panicking by now and wondering, "How in the world will I ever get by without ever eating anything deliciously sweet again?" The good news is that there are healthy alternatives that do not affect negatively impact your health.

Stevia is a non-caloric herbal sweetener that is perfectly safe and non-toxic. It can be used in baking and to sweeten your teas and lemonades. Some people find that the powdered Stevia has a bitter after taste while the liquid version is a little more palatable.

Another possible alternative to sugar are sugar alcohols, such as xylitol and erythritol. Although they contain much less sugar and

---

[78] http://www.ncbi.nlm.nih.gov/pmc/articles/PMC3267662/?tool=pubmed

require little or no insulin, they can contribute to slightly raising blood sugar levels. There has been some concern about the original source for the production of these sugar alcohols, as well as the chemicals that may be used to produce them. If you do use them, use them sparingly and occasionally.

Many women act surprised when I recommend the elimination of most grains from their diet. Grains, even the complex whole grains, eventually end up as glucose in the blood. A study conducted at the University of British Columbia, Canada, showed compelling proof of the ability of a low carbohydrate diet to slow down tumor growth and even prevent cancer initiation.[79] Using genetically engineered mice that are prone to mammary tumor development, the researchers noted that 50% of the mice that were fed a typical 'western diet' developed tumors, whereas no cancer was detected in mice being fed the low carbohydrate diet over the same period.

So no matter how you slice it, reduce, eliminate, and avoid all forms of sugar as much as possible.

GMO FOODS

If you want to prevent cancer or if you are on a healing journey with Breast Cancer, you must avoid GMO Foods. GMO foods create toxins and allergens that the body reacts to resulting in headaches, aching joints, and allergic reactions.

The World Health Organization has defined Genetically Modified Organisms (GMOs) as "organisms in which the genetic material (DNA) has been altered in such a way that does not occur naturally."

That should give you a clue. Historically, anytime man has fooled with Mother Nature, there have always been dire consequences.

A recent report, GMO Myths and Truths[80], authored by Dr. Michael Antoniou of Great Britain and Dr. John Harper of the US, provides evidence of peer-reviewed scientific studies about the hazards to

---

[79] http://www.ncbi.nlm.nih.gov/pubmed?term=21673053

[80] http://www.pakalertpress.com/2012/06/27/genetic-engineers-explain-why-ge-food-is-dangerous/

health and the environment posed by GMO foods. Feeding GMO foods to laboratory animals in feeding trials resulted in harmful effects including infertility, disruption of the immune system, rapid aging, issues with blood sugar regulation, as well as pathological effects to the liver, kidney, spleen, and digestive system.

Lastly, GMO cultivation has hurt our planet. Glyphosates are contaminating groundwater, the rivers, and lakes and are killing the healthy bacteria in the soil. Glycophosphates have been found in 60%-100% of all US air and rain samples, which means that even if you try to eat organic, you can thank chemical manufacturers for poisoning your food and air.

A great resource to learn more about the effects of GMO foods on your health can be found at www.nongmoproject.org. To ensure that you are not consuming GMO foods, always purchase food with the non-GMO label.

PROCESSED AND CHARRED MEATS

This can be a bit of a controversial topic. I have worked with women that were strictly vegan / vegetarian or some that were eating 100% raw. One might think that these raw foodists were faster healers and overcame challenges of Breast Cancer more quickly. However, I found that this has not always the case. Conversely, I have also consulted with women that included some animal protein in their diet along with a diet that was about 80% raw. In my opinion, these were the women that seem to respond much quicker to the suggested protocols.

A key concern of meat consumption is the byproducts that are produced when heating the meat at high temperatures:

- Heterocyclic amines (HCAs) (the charred, blackened meat).
- Polycyclic Aromatic Hydrocarbons (PAHs) (smoke from the dripping fat).
- Advanced Glycation End Products (AGEs) (cause oxidative stress).

All of these by-products of grilling meat at high temperatures have triggered the cancer process in laboratory animals.[81] Since grilling meat produces the highest amounts of carcinogens, cook it slowly and at lower temperatures to avoid the formation of the cancer causing chemicals.

Without getting into a complex explanation of some of the flaws in the China study that promotes 100% vegetarianism or the pros and cons of the meat-based Paleo diet, I would say that the most balanced approach is to create a diet that consists of 80% to 90% raw food with small portions of fish, beef, turkey, and chicken 3 to 4 times per week.

Personally, I have experimented with every type of diet known possible. When it came to my personal healing journey, I found that adding animal protein to my diet and eliminating carbs and sugars, allowed my body to function optimally. There is no cookie-cutter magic dietary cure. It comes down to balance and what works best for you.

If there's one thing I've learned in my 35 years in the wellness industry, is that some people thrive on a plant based diet while some thrive on a meat-based diet. The factors that influence this can be your blood type, your environment, your age, your previous health history, your metabolic type, and your body's ability to digest food effectively.

An example of an extreme meat-based diet is the Ketogenic Diet. This diet calls for replacing carbohydrates with healthy fats and oils and moderate amounts of high-quality protein. Healthy cells have the ability to use ketone bodies for energy rather than glucose, while cancer cells depend solely on glucose for energy. There have been studies and books written about the Ketogenic Diet[82] and the impact it had on breast, prostate, and brain cancers. Whether or not this diet is healthy long-term remains to be seen.

---

[81] http://preventcancer.aicr.org/site/News2?abbr=pr_&page=NewsArticle&id=13394&news_iv_ctrl=1102

[82] http://www.ncbi.nlm.nih.gov/pubmed/?term=ketogenic+diet+cancer

Obviously, if you're going to include meat in your diet, it must be antibiotic, hormone free, grass fed, grain free meat. Ideally, you should know the source of the meat by purchasing your meat from local markets and farmers. When you purchase fish make sure that it is wild caught and not farmed. The best fish to consume would be wild Pacific or Alaskan salmon.

DAIRY

Although there are massive campaigns that would have you believe that 'Milk Does the Body Good', homogenized and pasteurized dairy products are very toxic. And in plain terms, cow's milk is designed for baby cows, not humans. Thus, to support the growth of an animal that will eventually weigh about 1500 pounds, cow's milk has over 3 times the amount of protein (which is very difficult to digest) and 3 times the amount of calcium (which causes gall stones, kidney stones, and arthritic deposits.)

As human beings, we go through a natural weaning process that occurs between the ages of 5 to 7 years of age. ***Our body stops producing the lactase enzyme that breaks down the lactose or milk sugar. According to a study done in the 1970s, "Most of the world's human adults are lactose intolerant."***

Traditional store-bought milk is loaded with bovine growth hormones which are injected into the cows to increase their milk production. Injecting this hormone also increases the level of the insulin growth factor also known as IGF-I.

This increases the potential for Breast Cancer since the Insulin Growth Factor-I is a critical factor in stimulating tumor cells.[83]

Store-bought milk is loaded with pesticide residues and dioxins.

Dioxins are produced from the use of industrial chlorine, as well as paper bleaching and pesticide production. According to the World Health Organization, dioxins interfere with hormones that cause cancer. A study published in the *Journal of Clinical Oncology*

---

[83] http://www.ncbi.nlm.nih.gov/pubmed/8932606

recognized that milk and dairy products (as well as certain other food types) could increase the risk of Prostate cancer and other types of cancers.[84]

Some dairy advocates believe that as long as dairy products are consumed in the raw form, before pasteurization and homogenization, that they "do the body good." Milk is milk, no matter how you drink it. Obviously, drinking raw milk and consuming raw cheese is better than drinking or eating commercial dairy products. If you are on a healing journey with Breast Cancer or want to prevent Breast Cancer, I would encourage you to avoid dairy products of all kinds. An exception to that could be cultured dairy products such as plain yogurt or kefir.

I remember the day when replacing dairy products with organic nut milks was not as simple as picking up a quart from the local natural market. I used to make my almond milk and cashew milk from scratch. Now there are several varieties of nut milks that can be purchased. Purchase only the organic unsweetened variety of nut milks and coconut milk. Avoid rice milk because of the high sugar content.

WATER

Nothing is more important to sustaining our health than clean water. Since our body is made up of over 75% water, daily ingestion of clean water is vital to life. Water flushes impurities from our systems, helps to regulate body temperature, and regulates the digestive process.

First and foremost, ***do not drink tap water***. The World Health Organization has estimated that 75% to 80% of cancers may originate in our water and environment. The Environmental Working Group analyzed nearly 20,000,000 water samples between 2004 and 2009 and found over 316 contaminants in the water supply to the public.[85] These included agricultural pollutants, pesticides, chemicals and fertilizers, industrial chemicals from factories, as well as pollutants

---

[84] http://www.ncbi.nlm.nih.gov/pubmed/16278466
[85] http://www.ewg.org/tap-water/reportfindings.php

that were byproducts of the water treatment process itself. The majority of these chemicals are carcinogenic. Drinking tap water through your mouth and through your skin in the form of a shower subjects you to hundreds of chemicals in one sitting.

The onslaught of these chemicals in our water supply was responsible for creating a billion-dollar bottled water industry and water filtration industry. Unfortunately, bottled water has created its own problems.

In a test of the 10 best-selling brands of bottled water, the Environmental Working Group found over 38 different pollutants that included industrial chemical, fertilizers, and even bacteria.[86]

A study conducted by the Goethe University of Frankfurt found that the plastic bottles themselves were releasing estrogenic chemicals into the water. BPA or bisphenol A is a chemical compound that is used to make plastics and epoxy resins. This endocrine disrupting chemical has a direct effect on Breast Cancer development. Studies using cultures of human Breast Cancer cells have shown that BPA acts through the same pathways as estrogen. It has been shown to induce cell proliferation as well as DNA damage to human Breast Cancer cells.[87] With this in mind, do not purchase bottled water, unless it is stored in hard plastic that is BPA free.

When it comes to filtering your water, there are hundreds of choices. Your two best options are purchasing filters from Aqua Sauna[88] out of California or the Big Berkey[89] filter. (I personally prefer the convenience and efficiency of my Berkey!) For the cost, the Berkey filters provide you with the assurance that you are removing at least 99.999% of the toxins in tap water. Since you drink water through your skin when you shower or bathe, I highly recommend filters for your shower head and your bathtub faucet.

---

[86] http://www.ewg.org/news/news-releases/2011/01/05/what%E2%80%99s-your-bottled-water-%E2%80%93-besides-water

[87] http://www.breastcancerfund.org/clear-science/chemicals-glossary/bisphenol-a.html

[88] http://www.aquasana.com/

[89] http://breastcancerconquerorshop.com/product/berkey-water-filter/

How much water should you drink every day? The general rule is to drink half your weight in ounces of water. For example, if you weigh 150 pounds that you would drink approximately 75 ounces of pure clean water every day.

Under the subject of water, I must also mention filtration systems that also alkalize your water. I have heard testimonials from people who raved about their alkaline water but I've also talked to people who have developed serious digestive issues as a result of drinking alkaline water.

The theory behind drinking alkaline water is that it helps to alkalize an acidic body. Cancer cells thrive in an acidic environment and the idea of keeping the body alkaline with water sounds simple. However you must recognize that the stomach, by nature, is extremely acidic, with the pH of 2 or below. If too much alkaline water is consumed, this may create an issue with the pH of the stomach. If there's not enough acid in your stomach to properly digest your food, you're setting yourself up for many types of digestive health issues.

I once had a discussion with a gastroenterologist who promoted the use of alkaline water what he thought about the impact of alkaline water on the digestive system. He told me that he recommended the use of alkaline water certain times during the day: upon awakening, between meals, and before bed. Never was alkaline water to be ingested shortly before, after, or during meals, since the alkalinity could, in fact, interfere with proper digestion. If you feel that alkaline water is an important part of your healing journey, I encourage you to drink it wisely.

If you're really interested in alkalizing your water, the use of plain old simple baking soda can do the trick. 1 teaspoon of baking soda and 8 ounces of water can alkalize water to a pH of eight or nine. The same principles apply with the use of baking soda water as in alkaline water. Only drink a solution on an empty stomach and never with meals.

OILS

Buyer beware that there are some oils that are extremely toxic. Specific GMO oils such as canola oil, soybean oil, corn oil, and even sunflower oil should be avoided like the plague. They are cheap products to manufacture and are found in almost all processed and packaged foods and are labeled as trans-fats or hydrogenated fats.

Many of these oils have been found to deplete certain vitamins and interfere with enzyme function. Take the damage these oils do one step further by heating the oils at very high temperatures. There is a dangerous toxin called HNE (4- hydroxy-trans-2-nonenal) that is produced when polyunsaturated oils are heated at very high temperatures. This HNE causes lipid peroxidation on the cell wall which reduces cellular respiration.

The imbalances of too many omega 6 plant oils have promoted the pathogenesis of many diseases such as cancer, cardiovascular disease, and inflammatory autoimmune diseases. ***The healthiest combination of oils for Breast Cancer suppression would be found in the proper ratio of omega sixes and omega-3.***[90]

The *Journal of the National Cancer Institute* published a research paper about the effects of the proper ratio on Breast Cancer. They found that diets that were high in omega 6 actually stimulated the growth and spread of Breast Cancer cells. Conversely, they found that diets high in omega 3, such as fish oils, exerted a suppressive effect on Breast Cancer cells. The best source of omega-3 is from purified and distilled wild caught fish oil. Components of the fish oil, DHA and EPA, have an anti-inflammatory effect on cells and have also been shown to cause cell death to Breast Cancer cells.[91]

Other healthy sources for omega-3 oils can be found in flax seeds, chia, and hemp.

When purchasing cooking oils, the two best choices are organic, cold pressed grape seed oil and coconut oil which are sold in glass containers. Olive oil should not be used at a temperature higher than

---

[90] http://www.ncbi.nlm.nih.gov/pubmed/?term=12442909

[91] http://www.ncbi.nlm.nih.gov/pubmed/?term=14502842

150° since the high heat oil denatures the oil. Coconut oil and grape seed oils can be used for baking and cooking at high temperatures.

COFFEE

As much as you may like your morning cup of java, this is one daily beverage you should consider eliminating. Since our goal is to move your body towards alkalinity, eliminating daily consumption of coffee is an important step. There are, however, certain coffees that are roasted at very low temperatures which do not destroy the anti-oxidants in the coffee beans.[92] The processing retains the natural compounds found in the coffee beans that protect the stomach from distress.

You can replace your morning cup of coffee with some warm organic green tea. Green tea is loaded with anti-oxidants and catechins. Catechins (EGCG) are a type of anti-oxidant that halt oxidative damage to cells. Studies have shown that catechins suppress the growth, migrations, and invasion of human Breast Cancer cells.[93] The most powerful green tea is called Matcha Tea.[94]

One cup of Matcha Tea is equal to 10 cups of regular green tea.

I would recommend 2 cups per day. You can sweeten your tea with various forms of stevia-flavored drops.

Now let's move on to the foods that we can enjoy!

---

[92] https://www.levitamins.com/54692/ProductSearch?by=01730

[93] http://www.ncbi.nlm.nih.gov/pubmed/23646788

[94] http://www.shareasale.com/r.cfm?b=265885&u=839958&m=30043&urllink=&afftrack=

START FEEDING YOUR BODY

Now that we are pretty clear on what you need to avoid, let's focus on how much fun it can be to enjoy nourishing our bodies with powerful healing food. The very fact that you are clear about moving forward about nourishing your body with good food can be very motivational. Healthy food choices cannot be stressed enough. This is the foundation and building blocks that your cells use to either fight off the cancer or give in to it because they are too weak to resist.

I understand that food has many emotional connections attached to it. We associate good food with casual entertainment and time with family and friends. So what can we do to make this a joyful experience? It is all in your attitude.

If you constantly grieve the loss of your 'comfort foods' and keep wishing that you could keep eating them, then you are living in the past and are not taking full responsibility for your health. Remember that Breast Cancer did not just 'happen' to you. It came as a result of several factors, some for which you are ultimately responsible. Cancer cannot grow in a healthy body. So let's do whatever it takes to starve the cancer and feed your body.

THE ANDI SCORE

Dr. Joel Furhman, a board certified family physician and nutritional researcher, has coined the term, 'Nutritarian Eating' which focuses on a lifetime of a healthy intake of micronutrients. He has also created the ANDI scoring system which stands for: Aggregate Nutrient Density Index. The higher the rating on the food, the higher the concentration of micronutrients per calorie that are found in the food. You can learn more about this scoring system on his web site.[95] The top rating ANDI foods are found in the following list of 'The Top 7 Foods to Enjoy'.

Now the fun begins. You get to transform your health and vitality by adding new foods to your diet. You will be amazed at how simple

---

[95] http://www.drfuhrman.com/library/andi-food-scores.aspx

changes can make such a difference in the way you feel. You will want to balance your foods so that ultimately you are eating about 80% raw and 20% cooked. Why is raw so important?

Raw foods still have live enzymes that serve many functions. Enzymes are responsible for accelerating the rate of metabolic functions such as digestion and biological reactions in the cell. The average person consumes over 75% of their food in a cooked state; therefore, their body becomes enzyme deficient. We will talk about the use of adding enzyme therapy in Chapter 7, Essential #6: Repair Your Body.

THE TOP 7 FOODS TO ENJOY

CRUCIFEROUS VEGETABLES

Many of the chemicals that we are exposed to in our macro or micro environment can overwhelm and eventually block our detoxification pathways. Thankfully, Nature has supplied us with the most effective natural detoxifiers on the planet: cruciferous vegetables. Cruciferous vegetables optimize our Phase II detoxification system[96] in the liver, which helps to neutralize the effect these foreign chemicals have on our DNA.

In fact, if you increase your consumption of cruciferous vegetables, healthy oils, and specific low glycemic fruits, you can reduce your Breast Cancer risk by 60-70%.[97]

These cruciferous vegetables have been shown to control cancer's 'On and Off' switches in Breast Cancer.[98] But the most powerful cancer fighting component, glucosinolate, is found in broccoli and broccoli sprouts. These turn on protective genes[99], encourage cancer cell death, and turn off the genes that tend to promote cancer.

Cruciferous vegetable are especially important for women who are healing from Breast Cancer or want to prevent Breast Cancer. A study

---

[96] http://www.ncbi.nlm.nih.gov/pubmed/23110644
[97] http://www.nutritionj.com/content/pdf/1475-2891-3-19.pdf
[98] http://www.ncbi.nlm.nih.gov/pubmed/12873994
[99] http://www.ncbi.nlm.nih.gov/pmc/articles/PMC3042379/

by Vanderbilt-Ingram Cancer Center revealed that women who ate more cruciferous vegetables had an improved survival rate.[100]

The plant chemicals in cruciferous vegetables serve many functions:

- They alter estrogen metabolism[101]
- They prevent the spread of Breast Cancer to the lungs[102]
- They prevent the development of estrogen enhanced cancers, such as Breast, Cervical, and Endometrial[103]
- They reduce the risk of ever developing Breast Cancer[104]

Here is a list of the most common cruciferous vegetables:

- Arugula
- Kale
- Bok Choy
- Parsnips
- Broccoli
- Radishes
- Brussels sprouts
- Turnips
- Cabbage
- Watercress
- Cauliflower
- Wasabi

It is best to eat these raw, since cooking can destroy the powerful anti-cancer nutrients. Rather than trying to eat bowls and bowls of these raw vegetables, you can include them in your juicing and blending recipes. (More on this later.)

---

[100] http://www.mc.vanderbilt.edu/news/releases.php?release=2395

[101] http://en.wikipedia.org/wiki/Indole-3-carbinol

[102] http://www.ncbi.nlm.nih.gov/pubmed/19864400

[103] http://www.greenmedinfo.com/article/indole-3-carbinol-negative-regulator-estrogen

[104] http://www.ncbi.nlm.nih.gov/pubmed/22877795

The most potent phyto-chemicals can be found in the 3 day old Broccoli sprout, which contains around **50 times** more bioactivity than the mature plants. You can sprout your own quite easily or you can also buy the powdered concentrated form, Enduracell[105], from a company in Australia. These enzyme active sprouts yield a very high concentration of Sulforaphane.

Every woman on the planet should understand the power of Sulforaphane. Sulforaphane in broccoli sprouts has the following protective effects:[106]

- Turns on Phase II detoxification enzymes that protect against oxidative stress and promotes removal of cancer causing chemicals
- Suppresses cytochrome P450 enzymes
- Induces apoptotic pathways (cancer cell death)
- Suppresses cancer cell cycle progression
- Inhibits the formation of blood vessels that feed tumors (angiogenesis)
- Decreases inflammation

Now that you are aware of the power of the sprout[107], begin immediately by incorporating 2-3 servings of this in your diet. You can add the sprouts to your juicing and blending or you can add the powdered version just as easily. If you don't mind the taste of the sprout, you can mix it in water and drink within 15 minutes in order to keep the enzymes activity at its peak.

GREEN LEAFY VEGETABLES

Green leafy vegetables are highest on the ANDI score list. This includes:

---

105 http://breastcancerconquerorshop.com/product/broccoli-sprout-powder/

106 http://www.ncbi.nlm.nih.gov/pubmed/17396224?ordinalpos=9&itool=EntrezSystem2.PEntrez.Pubmed.Pubmed_ResultsPanel.Pubmed_DefaultReportPanel.Pubmed_RVDocSum

107 http://www.ncbi.nlm.nih.gov/pmc/articles/PMC23369/pdf/pq010367.pdf

- Kale
- Bok Choy
- Collard
- Greens
- Spinach
- Mustard
- Greens
- Parsley
- Watercress
- Romaine Lettuce
- Swiss Chard
- Arugula

Try to have at least 2 large servings of these every day. You can incorporate them in your salads or use several cups in your smoothies. It may seem boring to eat these same vegetables every day but if you get creative with the dressings and how you include them in your smoothies, you will find yourself craving them if you go a day without your greens.

A note about celery: although it is not considered a leafy green, it has many beneficial properties. A flavonoid called apigenin, which is found in celery and parsley, has been shown to inhibit the progression and development of Breast Cancer cells.[108] So make sure you include celery in your juicing and blending routines.

GREEN APPLES AND LEMONS

Since you are now aware that sugar feeds cancer, you want to minimize your intake of fruits while you are on your healing journey. The main fruits that you can enjoy while on your journey are green apples, lemons, and occasional berries.

---

[108] http://www.ncbi.nlm.nih.gov/pubmed/22569706

Green apples have the lowest sugar content of any of the apple categories and provide many anti-cancer benefits. Research conducted by The University of Wisconsin demonstrated the power of the apple peel.[109] An organic apple peel solution was dripped on petri dishes containing Breast Cancer cells and Prostate cancer cells. Both cancers eventually died off...with apple peels? Yep! "What was the mechanism that caused the cancer cells to die off?" you may ask?

There is a tumor suppressor gene called Maspin that is found in Breast and Prostate tissue. The cancer cells turn off that gene which allows the cancer cells to keep multiplying. Conversely, the phyto-chemicals in apple peels turn that protective gene back on. (More proof that your DNA is NOT your destiny.)

Data analyzed for over 10 years has proven that there is a consistent inverse association between apples and the risk for various cancers.[110]

An apple a day can keep the oncologist away!

When you enjoy your apples, always eat organic and eat the WHOLE apple, seeds included. Apple seeds contain the Vitamin B-17, which can form a natural barrier against cancer growth. When you juice the whole apple or blend it in a high powered blender like Vita-mix, you are getting the benefits of the peel and the seeds. Enjoy 1-2 green apples per day.

The next fruit that you can enjoy as much as you like are lemons. Lemons can be blended or juiced with your greens. I always start my day with the juice of 1 lemon in a glass of clean water. This serves to stimulate your digestive juices, wakes up your digestive system, and stimulates the liver and gall bladder.

The lemon peel and their extracts are loaded with potent flavonoids that have many health benefits and potent pharmacological activities.[111] These flavonoids have been proven to:

---

[109] http://youtu.be/KI-jaZTRU8M
[110] http://www.ncbi.nlm.nih.gov/pubmed/16091428
[111] http://www.ncbi.nlm.nih.gov/pubmed/23673480

- Down-regulate inflammatory enzymes
- Suppress the growth of tumors
- Slow down the spread of cancer cells
- Stop the growth of blood vessels that feed tumors
- Cause cancer cell death (apoptosis)

Specifically concerning Breast Cancer, the more citrus you eat, the lower your risk is for developing Breast Cancer.[112] In order to feed your body and starve the cancer, make it a goal to have at least 2 lemons per day.

NUTS AND SEEDS

Nuts are a rich source of nutrients such as Vitamin E, B2, folate, fiber, and essential minerals such as magnesium, selenium, and phosphorus. They are also a great source of Omega 3's and essential fatty acids. A handful of walnuts 3 times per week can help you meet the EFA requirements set by the WHO. ***Walnuts contain specific bioactive molecules that have shown beneficial effects in the prevention of Breast Cancer.***[113]

A couple of important facts about eating nuts:

- Always consume them raw.
- Always soak them overnight before eating them. Nuts have enzyme inhibitors to protect the seed or nut until it is in the right environment for growing. When you soak the nuts, the inhibiting enzymes are released and you begin the sprouting process for the nuts. The nuts then become a 'live' food and offer more nutritional value. They are also much easier to digest after they are soaked. You can air dry your nuts or place them in a dehydrator to speed up the process.
- They are relatively inexpensive and can be consumed as a snack or added to salads and main meals.

---

[112] http://www.ncbi.nlm.nih.gov/pubmed/23593085
[113] http://www.ncbi.nlm.nih.gov/pubmed/23061909

The best nuts to consume as part of your healing journey include:

- Almonds
- Pecans
- Brazil Nuts
- Pumpkin Seeds
- Cashews
- Sunflower Seeds
- Macadamian nuts
- Walnuts

No peanuts! They are loaded with fungal toxins and most are GMO.

Now let's talk about seeds, specifically Flax Seeds. When it comes to Breast Cancer, research has shown that flax seeds are one of the most beneficial foods you can consume. They are high in soluble and insoluble fiber and are the richest source of Omega 3 fatty acids.

A key component of flax seeds are lignans. ***Lignans are phytoestrogens (plant estrogens) which have estrogen-like qualities.*** They are also strong anti-oxidants. Now before you start to worry about the estrogen effect of flax seeds, let's look at the compelling research for the consumption of flax seeds.

- Dietary lignans reduce Breast Cancer risk by having a positive effect on estrogen signaling.
- Lignans have a protective effect against the more aggressive, proliferative estrogens.
- Flax seed extracts reduce Breast Cancer tumor growth.
- Flax seeds inhibit the spread of Breast Cancer.
- Flax Seeds inhibit the growth of estrogen-dependent Breast Cancer and even strengthened the effect of the toxic drug Tamoxifen.
- Flax seeds lower tumor markers in post-menopausal women. Breast Cancer patients at the University of Toronto, Canada, were asked to consume a muffin containing 25 grams of flaxseeds (about 5 teaspoons) for over 1 month. The result

clearly demonstrated that the women who consumed the muffins showed a decrease of tumor growth by 30% - 71%!

You can enjoy Flax Seeds by grinding them with a coffee grinder and sprinkling them on your salads, veggies, and in your smoothies. I have also soaked them, added a bit of flavoring, spread them on a sheet, and dehydrated them to make amazing crunchy raw crackers.[114]

Another important benefit of seeds and nuts are the high fiber content. If your diet is low in fiber and you have poor elimination, the estrogen that is broken down by the liver and sent to the colon to be eliminated will sit in the gut and be recirculated in your body. If there is plenty of fiber in your gut, the excess estrogen can be properly excreted. Fiber also helps to lower your Breast Cancer risk by regulating insulin and glucose metabolism. The higher the insulin levels, the greater your risk for developing Breast Cancer.

HEALTHY OILS

As previously discussed, the overuse of plant based oils for cooking, processing, and packaging has created diets that are too high in the Omega 6's and not enough of the Omega 3's. An imbalance in these ratios can lead to inflammation, cardiovascular disease, and other chronic illnesses.

Omega 3 fatty acids inhibit human Breast Cancer cell growth[115] and also decrease your risk[116] for developing Breast Cancer.

For healing purposes, let's focus on making sure we get plenty of Omega 3's.

Let's start with fish oils. There is a lot of controversy about the purity and safety of fish oils in capsule form. Sadly, most of the fish in our oceans and seas are contaminated with chemical pollutants and heavy metals such as mercury. Although many fish oils sold in capsule form have set high laboratory standards for distilling and 'purifying' the oil, in the end, is it really a healthy substitute for fresh fish? I have gone

---

114 http://breastcancerconqueror.com/raw-almond-bruschetta-crackers/
115 http://www.ncbi.nlm.nih.gov/pubmed/23285198
116 http://www.ncbi.nlm.nih.gov/pubmed/23137008

back and forth with this issue but ultimately I feel better if I focus on getting my healthy oils from clean fish such as wild caught salmon. If the fresh fish is not available, I will supplement about 3 times per week.

Healthy fats and oils include cold-pressed, extra virgin REAL olive oil, coconut oil, and grape seed oil. Olive oil should not be used to cook at high temperatures as this denatures the oil and will damage the Omega 3's.Olive oil is the better choice for salad dressings. Coconut oil and grape seed oil have a higher smoke point, so they are the better choice for cooking and baking.

Coconut oil is comprised of MCFAs or medium chain fatty acids. The fats are smaller than vegetable fatty acids and are easier to breakdown, increasing cell membrane permeability. Because of its metabolic effect, coconut oil increases the activity of the thyroid gland, which is absolutely critical if you are on a Breast Cancer healing journey.

Other sources of Omega 3's include: Flax seeds, walnuts, kidney beans, grass fed beef, and free range eggs.

By the way, a ¼ cup of ground Flax Seeds has over 3 times the amount of Omega 3's than a 4 ounce piece of salmon. So start grinding those flax seeds!

HEALTHY MEATS

For those of you who want to include a small amount of animal protein in your diet, there are a few absolutes:

- You know the source of your meat
- The animals are treated humanely
- The animals are hormone, antibiotic free
- They get to play outdoors and bask in the sun every day
- Their diet is 100% grass with no grain fillers

These factors will ensure that you have a healthy quality meat. Many of the studies that have been conducted on the pros and cons of a meat based diet versus a vegetarian diet have been based on grain fed, slaughter house meats. You may be surprised to learn the benefits of grass fed beef:

- High in Omega 3's
- The richest source of CLA, conjugated linoleic acid, which is a powerful anticarcinogen
- In a Finnish study, higher levels of CLA in the blood were associated with a lower Breast Cancer risk
- Higher in Vitamin E

Some metabolic types may be better suited for a vegetarian diet, where as some others may improve their healing when they include small amounts of animal protein.

What exactly does 'small amounts of animal protein' mean? A small serving, no bigger than a deck of cards, and not necessarily every day. To ensure proper digestion of the meat, implementing digestive enzymes and betaine HCl with every meal is important.

Fermented Foods

The S.A.D. diet and the overuse of antibiotics have left most people with unhealthy guts which have become a breeding ground for unhealthy bacteria, fungi, viruses, and parasites. The toxins from the environment are not properly eliminated, leading to serious problems with leaky gut syndrome and other chronic health issues.

Fermented foods date back to Egyptian times. Evidence of fermented foods has been found in most ancient cultures around the globe. Fermented foods are rich in enzymes, improve digestion, and help to restore the proper bacterial flora in the gut.

The best types of fermented foods are:

- Kefir, preferably coconut milk or goat milk based.
- Real yogurt, preferably coconut milk or goat milk based.
- Raw sauerkraut and other fermented vegetables.
- Miso, a fermented soybean paste can be used as a soup broth. Do not boil as this will kill the active enzymes and bacteria.

- Kombucha, which is high in glucoronic acid, which assists liver detoxification.

I typically have at least 1 serving of a fermented food every day. My favorites are Kombucha and coconut milk Kefir.

So there you have it.

You have learned about the top 7 foods that you must avoid in order to stop feeding the cancer and the top 7 foods that you can enjoy that will nourish your body.

So how do you put all of this together in a practical day to day lifestyle? Great question!

Before I provide you with a real-life daily menu as well as practical steps for our Pantry Swap, let's discuss the many fashionable and popular diets.

WHICH DIET IS RIGHT FOR ME?

I'll be the first to admit that the plethora of diets that are out there can be very confusing for the average consumer. There are literally over 100 different diets that claim to be the next miracle cure. *The key is to find the right balance for you.* The most important factor to remember in choosing a dietary lifestyle is that you want to feed and nourish your body and starve the cancer.

After many years of experimenting with various ways of eating, one question that I ask myself before I put anything in my body is this: "Will this help or hinder my body?"

Do I have the perfect diet? No. Do I occasionally cheat with coffee, bread, a glass of wine, and occasional dessert? Yes. But overall, I am very conscious about what I put in my body.

These are the diets that I have experimented with over the last 35 years:

- Adkins
- Blood type diet
- Budwig Diet

- Fasting and Cleansing Diets
- Ketogenic Diet
- Macrobiotics
- Mediterranean Diet
- Raw food only
- Vegetarian
- Vegan

I have not experimented with the Gerson Diet simply because, for me, I find there are too many sugars in all the juices. Personally, 4 + coffee enemas per day for an extended period of time seems to be excessive.

BLENDING AND JUICING

Juicing involves grinding, pulverizing, and squeezing the juices out of specific fruits and vegetables. The benefit of juicing, especially if you are having some serious challenges with your health, is that you can absorb more nutrients with less effort. The juices are absorbed more quickly into the bloodstream, allowing the digestive system to rest. If you want to overcome the side effects of traditional cancer treatments such as chemo and radiation, juicing may be your beverage of choice for several months.

Blending has become very popular with kitchen aids as the Vitamix and the Nutribullet blender and is often referred to as 'smoothies. This method grinds and breaks down leafy vegetables so they are more easily assimilated. You can 'eat' more greens if you blend them, instead of sitting there trying to eat plate after plate of salads.

Blending drinks oxidize less quickly than juicing drinks. Since green leaves are not starchy, you can add a green apple and a lemon, without any bloating or digestive issues. You can also add flax seeds, chia seeds, and raw whey protein[117] to increase your glutathione production.

---

[117] http://breastcancerconquerorshop.com/product/one-world-whey-vanilla-1-lb/

A great resource for blending basics and recipes is *Greens for Life*[118] by Vitoria Boutenko.

So back to the original question: which diet is right for me? Make it a matter of Conscious Eating.

Conscious Eating is a new way of looking at your food. It is about making food choices that will support the healing and hinder the cancer. You have full responsibility.

You get to decide if you want to feed the cancer or feed your body...you pick.

Unfortunately, too many people dig their graves with their forks by making choices based on immediate gratification and food addictions.

Conscious Eating involves being thankful for the food that is on your plate and visualizing the food being digested properly and vibrantly nourishing your cells.

Conscious Eating recognizes the fact that everything is energy...our bodies, the food we eat, and the water we drink. Blessing your food with love and gratitude adds to the enjoyment and the benefit of your meal.

After we do our Pantry Swap, I will share a sample 7 Day Breast Cancer Healing Diet.

LET'S DO A PANTRY SWAP

TV celebrities are swapping wives, kids, and homes. But we are going to keep it simple and simply swap out the toxic, cancer feeding foods, with simple, organic, vibrant foods.

There is no need to go into panic mode and wonder how in the world are you going to change so many things all at once? I do know of women who have thrown everything out of their cupboards and started fresh. They were determined and ready to start the healing journey. Others, because of their budget, simply replaced their old products with organic ones, as they ran out of things.

---

118 http://www.rawfamily.com/products

Changing your eating habits is not as difficult as it seems. If you have certain foods that you really enjoy, chances are you'll be able to find a very healthy replacement. Let's take pasta for example. We all love our carbohydrate fix with cheesy tomato pasta. Do you know that you can purchase pasta that is made with black beans, mung beans, or quinoa?

Here is a basic check list for you so you can eventually turn your kitchen into an organic, life promoting kitchen.

Replace these Cancer Triggers with these Anti-cancer Exchanges.

- Replace sugar of all types with Stevia and sugar alcohols.
- Replace GMO foods with organic, non-GMO foods.
- Replace canned foods with BPA free, canned organic foods.
- Replace regular milk and dairy products with unsweetened, organic nut milks.
- Replace regular cheeses with organic, raw, grassfed goat, sheep or nut milk cheeses.
- Replace regular sweetened yogurt with organic, plain yogurt or kefir.
- Replace tap or bottled water with purified and filtered water.
- Replace roasted coffees and teas with organic Matcha tea and herbal teas.
- Replace store bought salad dressings with homemade dressings made with olive oil and lemon.
- Replace roasted and salted nuts with organic, raw, soaked nuts.
- Replace lard and margarine with organic coconut oil or grapeseed oil.
- Replace butter with grassfed, pasture raised organic butter.
- Replace peanut, corn, safflower, canola oils with organic, cold-pressed olive or coconut oil.
- Replace store bought commercial meats with pasture raised, grass fed local meats.
- Replace sodas with kombucha or sparkling mineral water.

- Replace wheat flour with almond flour.
- Replace rice with quinoa or millet.
- Replace wheat crackers with almond, gluten free crackers.
- Replace potato chips with kale chips or sprouted bean chips.
- Replace regular corn chips with organic, certified, non-GMO corn chips.
- Replace peanut butter with raw almond or sunflower seed butter.
- Replace white table salt with Himalayan Crystal salt.
- Replace chocolate bars and candy with organic, sugar-free, dark chocolate.

SEVEN DAY ANTI-CANCER SAMPLE MENU

Here is an example of a very simple menu for you to follow and guide you over the next seven days. Remember that you want to nourish the body and starve the cancer.

I always start my day with the juice of 1 lemon in a glass of water, probiotics, Beta Glucans, enzymes, and sublingual B-12. For an occasional indulgence, enjoy a piece of a dark chocolate, sweetened with Stevia. ☺

DAY 1

For Breakfast, enjoy at least 16 ounces of a Green Juice.

For Lunch, enjoy at least 16 ounces of a Green Smoothie.

For Dinner, enjoy Chicken Soup and a Broccoli salad.

Snacks can be a mixture of raw, soaked almonds or pecans.

Throughout the day, sip on Chaga tea, Matcha tea, Essiac Tea, or Lemon water.

DAY 2

For Breakfast, enjoy a homemade Almond flour muffin with a poached egg.

For Lunch, enjoy at least 16 ounces of a Green Juice.

For Dinner, enjoy a baked Organic chicken with sautéed broccoli, garlic and onions.

Snacks can be raw almond or flax crackers topped with raw almond butter or hummus.

Throughout the day, sip on Chaga tea, Matcha, Essiac Tea, and Lemon water.

DAY 3

For Breakfast enjoy at least 16 ounces of a Green Juice.

For Lunch, you can enjoy at least 16 ounces of a Green Smoothie.

For Dinner, you can enjoy wild-caught salmon with a Caesar or spinach salad.

Snacks can be celery sticks with almond butter and apricot kernels.

Throughout the day sip on Chaga tea, Matcha, Essiac Tea and Lemon water.

DAY 4

For Breakfast you can enjoy homemade Flax bread and 16 ounces of Green Juice.

For Lunch, mix up the Budwig mixture with blueberries and nuts with a small salad on the side.

For Dinner you can enjoy a bowl of grass fed beef broccoli stew.

Snack can be a green apple topped with almond butter.

Throughout the day sip on Chaga tea, Matcha, Essiac Tea and Lemon water.

DAY 5

For Breakfast, enjoy at least 16 ounces of a Green juice.

For Lunch, enjoy an avocado salad with 1 hard-boiled egg.

For Dinner, enjoy 4 ounces of Salmon with a spinach and baby kale salad.

Snacks can be raw almond dip with raw vegetable sticks.

Throughout the day sip on Chaga tea, Matcha, Essiac Tea, and Lemon water.

DAY 6

For Breakfast enjoy at least 16 ounces of a Green Smoothie.

For Lunch, enjoy a raw vegetable soup with an almond biscuit.

For Dinner, enjoy baked Cod with sautéed broccoli and veggies.

Snack can be an indulgence of a home-made raw apple pie.

Throughout the day sip on Chaga tea, Matcha, Essiac Tea, and Lemon water.

DAY 7

For Breakfast, enjoy at least 16 ounces of a Green juice.

For Lunch, enjoy a Spinach salad with baked wild-caught salmon or baked chicken.

For Dinner, enjoy a Quinoa broccoli casserole topped with flax seeds and sprouted nuts.

Snacks can be raw, soaked, sunflower seeds or pecans.

Throughout the day sip on Chaga tea, Matcha, Essiac Tea, and Lemon water.

After completing this chapter, you are light years ahead of so many women when it comes to healing Breast Cancer. Congratulations on getting this far! Keep it light, fun, and be adventurous as you learn to balance your food choices. You will find delicious Delectable Dishes[119] with all kinds of enjoyable recipes on my web site. Healthy eating gets easier because you will feel better physically and emotionally, knowing that you are taking positive steps in starving the cancer and nourishing your body.

POINTS TO PONDER

- I can starve the cancer or nourish my body with my food choices.
- Cancer loves acidic food and thrives in an acidic environment.
- Sugar of ANY kind feeds the cancer.
- GMO foods are toxic and result in harmful effects to the body.
- Commercial store bought meat is grain fed (with many other toxic fillers) and is loaded with hormones and antibiotics.
- Grass fed meats and eggs have higher levels of Omega 3's and CLA.
- Mass produced dairy products have growth hormones that lead to various cancers.
- Tap water has hundreds of cancer causing chemicals in it.
- There are too many toxic oils in the S.A.D.
- The ANDI score helps me to identify the top nutrient dense foods.
- Cruciferous vegetables supply strong detoxification nutrients that help to metabolize estrogen.
- 2 apples a day may keep the oncologist away.
- Raw nuts should be soaked before eating.
- 5 teaspoons of ground flax seeds may reduce your tumor markers.
- Fermented foods fill your gut with healthy bacteria.

---

119 http://breastcancerconqueror.com/delectable-dishes/

- Blending and juicing are an excellent way to increase my raw vegetable intake.

Your Healing Journey Action Steps

- Purchase 3 types of organic Cruciferous Vegetables and incorporate them in your menu for the week.
- Purchase 3 of the top organic Green Leafy Vegetables and incorporate them in your menu for the week.
- If you have a high powered blender, experiment with some blending recipes. You can find a few of my favorites on my web site
- Start your morning with a large glass of water and the juice of an organic lemon. You can also add 1 tsp. of baking soda to really alkalize your body. Wait at least 30 minutes before eating anything.
- Soak a cup of organic almonds overnight. Drain the next morning. Let air dry or dehydrate. Enjoy these as a snack throughout the day.
- Grind 5 teaspoons of flax seeds in the morning. Add them to your smoothie or sprinkle on your salads and veggies.
- Purchase organic, cold pressed coconut oil and use it from this day forward for cooking or baking. You can also use grape seed oil.
- Make your salad dressings with extra-virgin, cold-pressed olive oil and lemon juice.
- Find out where you can purchase grass fed, antibiotic and hormone free meats and eggs.
- Purchase Kefir and Kombucha. Stick with those that have the lowest sugars. GT's Kombucha has 2 grams of sugar per serving. You can also learn to make your own kefir and Kombucha.
- Focus on having 2 raw meals per day. A meal can be 2 large glasses of fresh vegetable juice or a blended vegetable drink.

- Drink half your weight in ounces of water. Write it down here so you will remember how much to drink every day.
- My weight_________ divided by 2 = ________ ounces I commit to drinking every day
- I am slowly converting my kitchen to a healthy living kitchen with The Pantry Swap.
- I commit to trying the sample 7 Day Anti-Cancer Menu. It's OK if I don't follow it 100%. Simply incorporating 1 or 2 of those meals per day can make a huge difference in my health.
- Write down how you are feeling about changing your diet. Is it hard? Are you resistive to the change? Do you miss certain comfort foods? Gently remind yourself that sometimes change can be challenging. You don't have to make a perfect transition all at once. Be positive about making a conscious choice about your food: Starve the cancer and nourish your body.

CHAPTER 3

ESSENTIAL #2 - REDUCE YOUR TOXIC EXPOSURE

"Take care of your body. It's the only place you have to live."

~

Jim Rohn

WHAT IS A TOXIN?

A toxin is a poisonous substance. It can be produced within living cells and organisms or created by man-made chemicals. I believe you can agree that we live in an environmentally toxic world that has impacted our health and the future of this planet.

Over 77,000 chemicals are produced in North America every year.[120] There are over 3000 chemicals added to our food supply. There are over 10,000 chemicals used in the food processing industry and most of them have never been tested for safety. Over 10,000 new chemicals are introduced each year. These chemicals are responsible for severe

---

120 http://www.nativevillage.org/Messages%20from%20the%20People/How%20to%20avoid%20environmental_toxins.htm

neurological disorders, hormonal imbalances, and Immune System disorders, including cancer.

Heather White, executive director of the Environmental Working Group, recently informed a Senate House hearing, "Under current law, chemical manufacturers can market new chemicals without giving federal regulators a safety test."[121] Scary but true!

In order to learn how to reduce your toxic exposure, I am going to break down all the various ways that we are exposed to toxins, how they affect us, and what you can do to protect your environment, your home, and your body from this assault of poisons.

ENVIRONMENTAL TOXINS

The United States imports or produces 42 billion pounds of chemicals *per day!* I don't know about you, but it is difficult for me to wrap my brain around that very concept! Over 10 years ago, the CDC conducted a national survey by analyzing the blood and urine of participants all over the U.S. They found that the average person had a total of 212 foreign chemicals in their blood, urine, and saliva.

How does our body handle the onslaught of these chemicals? What effect do these chemicals have on our Immune System and detoxification pathways? I am in awe of the body's ability to adapt to this toxic soup that it inadvertently ingests every day.

ENVIRONMENTAL LINKS TO BREAST CANCER

Becoming a conscious consumer is a first step in reducing your toxic exposure. Chemicals that are carcinogenic mean that they can alter the DNA to cause cancer or that they cause cells to multiply more rapidly which eventually leads to cancer. A growing body of evidence and research indicates that there is a connection between the development of Breast Cancer and environmental toxins.

---

[121] http://www.ewg.org/release/ewg-tells-congress-most-chemicals-market-aren-t-tested-safety

- Over 70 % of Breast Cancers have no known risk factors such as having children later in life or family history of Breast Cancer. That means that the high percentile of Breast Cancers is associated with environmental factors.
- Industrialized countries have higher incidences of Breast Cancer.
- Many industrial chemicals are Xeno-estrogens or false estrogens but mimic estrogen in the body, which increases the risk of Breast Cancer.

The list of chemicals having an estrogenic effect is very long. In fact, if you go to this link[122] for the American Cancer Society, you will find pages and pages of cancer causing chemicals.

You may be surprised to find Tamoxifen and X-ray radiation categorized as carcinogenic!

Here are the major groups of chemicals that have estrogenic effects on your body:

- Pesticides which includes insecticides, herbicides, and fungicides
- Any products associated with plastics including BPA in canned foods
- Chemicals in the water supply from detergents and surfactants
- Industrial chemicals such as dioxins, PCBs, and benzene derived products
- Estrogenic drugs that are in the water supply

So how does one escape the effect of these chemicals as they are everywhere in our environment? Begin by protecting your small corner of the planet: your yard and your home.

- Avoid the use of artificial lawn fertilizers and herbicides.
- Don't drink bottled water, especially if it has been sitting in the sun.

---

122 http://www.cancer.org/cancer/cancercauses/othercarcinogens/generalinformationaboutcarcinogens/known-and-probable-human-carcinogens

- Never use the microwave and cook your food in plastic containers.
- Purchase a reliable water filtering system for your drinking and bathing.
- Try to eat only organic food. If that is not possible, peel the fruit and vegetables that have been commercially produced.

ENVIRONMENTAL RADIATION – CELL PHONES, TOWERS, AND SATELLITES

This was a huge piece of the puzzle that I had personally missed when it came to my personal healing journey. Through bio-energetic testing, I discovered that I was very 'electro-sensitive to EMFs. Once I learned how to use my cell phone wisely and discovered ways to protect myself from all the EMFs in the air, I felt a tremendous amount of physical and mental relief.

If you live in a metropolitan area, take a look around you as you drive down the interstate. You will see massive cell towers and transmitters on hotel and corporate buildings.

If you want to know how many cell towers that are in your area, simply visit antennasearch.com and put in your city, state, and zip code.[123] Sometimes it takes a few minutes to process depending on how many towers there are, so be patient. You will discover the number of cell towers and antenna within a 4 mile radius of your home or business.

I will use the City of Atlanta for example. If you are standing in the downtown area on 14th street, you are surrounded by 870 antenna and 104 cell towers within a 2 mile radius! Add to that all the WI-FI hot spots and cell phone communication and you are literally swimming in a smog of EMFs.

You and I are electrical beings that function because of the bio-electrical signals from our brain, nerve system, and heart. Chronic environmental exposures to EMFs from cell phones, WI-FI, and

---

123 http://antennasearch.com/

satellite can have an impact on this delicate transmission system in our body. Radio Frequency Radiation (RFR) has skyrocketed as a result of cell tower sites being placed in school grounds and neighborhoods.

The most pervasive and invasive components of Electro-pollution are the new 'smart-meters'. Every home and building that once had an electric meter to measure the usage of electricity is being replaced with a wireless device that communicates with the electrical company's home base. These devices produce constant spikes of EMF exposure to millions of home and office buildings. In spite of adverse health effects, health concerns from experts, and much public pressure, the smart meters are growing in numbers.

Now before you start dismissing the idea of non-ionizing radiation from cell phones and cell towers having an effect on your health, let's take a look at the facts that have been validated by scientists around the world.

The Bio-initiative Report[124] was prepared by 29 scientists from all over the world, independent of any government agencies and industrial societies. They are doctors and Ph.D. s that are concerned about the effects of Electro-pollution on the planet, the people, and especially unborn children and young children.

They have spent years studying the data and thousands of research papers. They have no monetary gain in publishing the truth about this perilous toxin. The 2012 conclusion Bio-Initiative Report sends a clear message:[125]

Bio-effects are clearly established and occur at very low levels of exposure to electromagnetic fields and radiofrequency radiation.

Bio-effects can occur in the first few minutes at levels associated with cell and cordless phone use.

---

124 http://www.bioinitiative.org/

125 http://www.bioinitiative.org/report/wp-content/uploads/pdfs/section_1_table_1_2012.pdf

Bio-effects can also occur from just minutes of exposure to mobile phone masts (cell towers),WI-FI, and wireless utility 'smart' meters that produce whole body exposure.

Chronic base station level exposures can result in illness.

Reported Biological Effects from Cell Tower, WI-FI, Wireless laptops, and smart meters:[126]

- The production of stress proteins
- Disrupted Immune System
- Oxidative damage to the cell
- DNA damage
- Disrupted Calcium Metabolism
- Brain Tumors
- Weakened blood-brain barrier (This is the filter that protects your brain from toxins)
- Sleep problems
- Memory problems
- Learning and behavior problems
- Cancer and cell proliferation
- Cardiac, heart muscle, blood pressure, and vascular effects
- Reproductive disorders and fertility effects

Were you aware of the fact that the World Health Organization has examined the new health studies and data and has classified cell phone and cordless phone radiation as a possible human carcinogen?[127] This is the same category as lead and DDT.

When you hold a cell phone to your head, you are radiating the most important part of your body – your brain! It is not speculation any more, since studies have shown that this produces 'hot spots' in the

---

[126] http://www.bioinitiative.org/report/wp-content/uploads/pdfs/BioInitiativeReport-RF-Color-Charts.pdf

[127] http://ehtrust.org/leading-epidemiologists-conclude-that-cell-and-cordless-phone-radiation-is-a-probable-human-carcinogen/

brain. Other than the possibility of developing a brain tumor, EMFs from cell phones and other wireless devices suppress the production of Melatonin. Melatonin is widely known as the 'sleep hormone' but did you realize that melatonin is classified as a cytotoxin and tumor suppressor? Melatonin actually puts Breast Cancer cells to sleep.[128]

But if the effect this radiation has on your brain is not worrisome enough, the plume of radiation from the cell phone extends about 3 feet. So think about the other organs you may be radiating: your thyroid, heart, and breasts. There is a serious connection with hypothyroidism and Breast Cancer, which we will discuss in Chapter 7, Essential #6 – Repair Your Body.

I realize that I have discussed Electro-pollution in Chapter 1, and I am bringing it up again because it is a serious problem that you must be aware of. You may not see the EMFs in the air, but if you could, it would be like heavy dark smog that permeates the very space we live in. ***If the radiation from a cell phone can travel through a cement wall when you are in a building, do you think it is possible that that same radiation is traveling through your body?***

To learn more about this technology and its benefits, visit GIA Wellness.[129] Personally, my home, my electronic devices, and my body are all fully protected with this amazing technology.

ENVIRONMENTAL TOXINS IN OUR FOOD SUPPLY

Although I have discussed dietary Cancer Triggers in the previous chapter, there are a few more points that need to be made concerning food and learning to reduce your toxic exposure.

The Environmental Working Group has compiled a list of foods called the Dirty Dozen and the Clean Fifteen[130] that reflect the worst conventional foods to eat as well as the least toxic foods. Since pesticides are very potent Xeno-estrogens, it is important to pay attention to the foods that have the highest pesticide residues.

---

128 http://tulane.edu/news/releases/12112008_pr.cfm
129 http://www.giawellness.com/drveronique/products/terra-gia/
130 http://www.ewg.org/foodnews/

The USDA and FDA conducted studies on conventional crops and found that:[131]

- 98% of apples hade detectable levels of pesticides
- 42 different pesticide residues were found on domestic blueberries
- 78 different pesticides were found on lettuce samples
- 64 different pesticides were found on grapes

A few of the cleanest foods are avocados, cabbage, onions, and sweet peas. If you are serious about becoming more conscious about your food choices and the toxins in your environment, please visit their web site.[132]

If you like fish, there are certain fish that you will want to avoid because of the contamination of heavy metals such as mercury and lead and industrial chemicals such as PCBs and pesticides. The Environmental Defense Fund has a great web site that gives you a list about the best and worst choices of fish to eat.[133]

Canned foods are basically dead food. I have seen gas spectrometry pictures of canned food, and there is no life energy being emitted from the food. Canned foods are lined with a chemical resin called BPA or Bispenol A. Studies have shown that BPA has a direct effect on Breast Cancer cells because of its estrogenic properties.[134] It causes DNA damage and induces cellular proliferation in breast cells. There are products that are labeled BPA-free but unfortunately many of the replacements are more genotoxic than BPA itself.[135]

---

[131] http://www.ewg.org/news/news-releases/2012/06/19/ewg-releases-2012-shopper%E2%80%99s-guide-pesticides-produce

[132] http://www.ewg.org/

[133] http://seafood.edf.org/guide/best

[134] http://www.breastcancerfund.org/clear-science/chemicals-glossary/bisphenol-a.html

[135] http://www.greenmedinfo.com/blog/corporations-replace-bpa-more-dna-damaging-bisphenols?utm_source=GreenMedInfo+Weekly&utm_campaign=f11e9b0d29-Greenmedinfo&utm_medium=email&utm_term=0_62bb7ef31e-f11e9b0d29-86936749

Plastic containers and plastic wraps should also be avoided. They contain BPA and phthalates that are plastic softeners. The best plastic is no plastic but if you must use some, make sure they are marked with a #1, #2, #4 or #5.[136] These do not contain BPA.

NEVER use the microwave and NEVER eat anything that has been microwaved in a plastic container. The heat breaks down the chemicals and releases the toxins into your food.

Styrofoam cups and plates should be thrown out right away. Styrene, the chemical that is used to make Styrofoam, has been shown to deplete glutathione, which is a primary anti-oxidant that protects against free radical damage. It causes DNA damage and has shown evidence of estrogenic properties. According to a report by the National Toxicology Program, "Styrene could put some individuals at higher risk for carcinogenicity."[137] Styrofoam is especially dangerous when the food or liquid is hot.

HOUSEHOLD TOXINS

I have already discussed the toxins that affect your outdoor home space so now it is time to move indoors. The EPA has estimated that the quality of air on our homes can be 5 to 100 times more toxic than outdoor air. There are many sources of indoor air pollution in most homes that can lead to respiratory diseases, heart disease, and cancer:[138]

- Heating products such as oil, gas, kerosene, coal, or wood.
- New building materials, new furniture, and new carpeting that emit formaldehyde and other noxious chemicals. Formaldehyde is a pungent smelling gas that can cause respiratory irritations, and it is a 'probable carcinogen'.
- Commercial cleaning products: The average household has between 3 to 25 gallons of toxic cleaning products. The most

---

136 http://www.ewg.org/research/healthy-home-tips/tip-3-pick-plastics-carefully

137 http://ntp.niehs.nih.gov/NTP/roc/twelfth/2010/FinalBDs/Styrene_Final_508.pdf#search=styrofoam

138 http://www.epa.gov/iaq/ia-intro.html

dangerous chemicals are 'ethylene based glycols' that are used in floor cleaners, paints, plastics, and in synthetic fibers. A 2008 European study found that inhalation of these chlorine based compounds could "significantly increase the cancer risk". Cleaning products that contain bleach (floor cleaners, dishwasher detergents, clothing detergents, and bathroom cleaners) and similar disinfectants can react to create volatile chlorinated compounds.

- Pesticide sprays.
- Artificial candles, scented sprays, and fragrances are made from Volatile Organic Compounds. Many of the VOCs in your home are known carcinogens and should be avoided. It's difficult to really know what is in the fragrances, since the FDA does not require that the manufacturers disclose the chemicals in their fragrances. A recent study found 10 VOCs in common air fresheners and laundry products that were designated toxic by the EPA. So if any of your products have that 'fresh mountain air' scent or 'pumpkin pie scent', you are breathing VOCs.
- Dry Cleaning Chemicals: That sweet smell that lingers in your clothes after you have them dry cleaned is called PERC or perchloro-ethylene. It is an effective cleaning solvent but is a 'likely human carcinogen'. PERC has caused cancer in laboratory animals whether they inhaled it or ingested it. If you do dry clean your clothes, it has been suggested that you air out your clothes in the garage or outdoor back porch for at least 24 hours.
- Mercury vapors from CFL light bulbs: There is NO safe level of mercury. It is the most toxic metal on the planet. I spent years detoxing mercury out of my body because of amalgams, so I personally choose to not bring anything into my home that contains mercury. What happens if you break a CFL light bulb? The EPA tells you to leave the room, open windows, and shut off the AC or heating system so as to not spread the vapors. Sounds too risky for me!

- Nonstick cookware is manufactured with a chemical called PFOA or C8. It is found in the blood in the general US population, and it causes adverse effects to laboratory animals. It is an endocrine disruptor and has estrogenic effects. Quick heating like stir frying in a non-stick pan can release up to 6 cancer causing gases into your home environment. PFOA is also used in 'wrinkle-free' clothing, carpeting, and microwave popcorn packaging.
- Aluminum cookware and aluminum foils are very reactive, and the metal can leach into your food. Aluminum absorption has been associated with neurodegenerative diseases. Never wrap your food in aluminum foil or cook with aluminum foil.
- Molds can produce spores that float in the air. These molds can cause allergic reactions and suppress the Immune System.

DETOX YOUR HOME

At first it may seem overwhelming but if you take it one step at a time, you can detox your home environment and make it a healthier and safer haven. The best place to start is with your cleaning products. There are many companies that offer safer and healthier alternatives for your cleaning supplies. Check out the Environmental Working Group's web site[139] for a list of safe cleaning supplies. Ava Anderson Non Toxic[140] has very clean and simple cleaning products that are non-toxic or harmful to the environment.

Pesticides can easily be replaced with safe nontoxic substances. To learn how to do this you can read an article I wrote for Natural News.com: NonToxic Pest Control.[141]

Here is a simple check list you can use to start reducing your toxic exposure in your home. Simply check off the box when you have eliminated one of the products. You will see yourself making progress

139 http://www.ewg.org/key-issues/consumer-products/cleaning-products
140 http://www.avaandersonnontoxic.com/drv
141 http://breastcancerconqueror.com/non-toxic-pest-control/

before you know it. Even 1 check mark is a great step in the right direction.

- Cleaning Products
- Dish Soap
- Dusting Sprays
- Dish washing machine soap
- Regular floor cleaner
- Bathroom cleansers
- Chlorinated Products
- Detergents
- Dryer sheets
- Cookware
- Aluminum pots and pans
- Aluminum baking sheets
- Aluminum foil used to cook
- Microwave oven
- Nonstick cookware
- Plastic containers and utensils
- Fragrances
- Artificially scented candles
- Air fresheners
- Scented sprays
- Dry Cleaning chemicals
- Mercury CFL light bulbs
- Pesticide sprays and products

EXTERNAL TOXINS

The US government does not require any health studies or pre-market testing of the chemicals that are used in personal care products. There are over 10,000 chemicals used in personal care products and only 11 of these have been rejected as unsafe. The average person applies 15 or more products per day which exposes them to over 127 unique chemicals each day.[142]

LOTIONS AND POTIONS:

You are what you eat....whether it enters your mouth or is delivered through your skin. Because of the vast supply of capillaries in the skin, any substance that is applied to the skin inevitably ends up in the blood stream. If you apply a lotion to your skin, you are 'eating' the lotion through the skin.

How much lotion are you eating per day?

If you apply 1 tablespoon of lotion on your skin every day for 5 years, you would end up 'eating' over 7 gallons of toxic lotion.

If that lotion contains silicone derived ingredients, petroleum by products, chemical fragrances, and artificial dyes, then you are subjecting your body to gallons of toxins that can potentially accumulate in your liver, colon, and fatty cells.

The chemicals in lotions are toxic[143] to the reproductive system, affect the hormone system, and are known or suspected carcinogens. Shaving creams would also fall into this category.

There are too many chemicals to list but here a few major ones to avoid. For a more comprehensive list visit EWG's Skin Deep Cosmetic Database.[144]

- Artificial dyes and coal tar ingredients: human carcinogen.
- BHA: a preservative that causes cancer.

---

142 http://www.ewg.org/skindeep/2011/04/12/why-this-matters/
143 http://www.ewg.org/skindeep/2011/04/12/why-this-matters/
144 http://www.ewg.org/skindeep/

- DMDM: a preservative that releases formaldehyde, which causes cancer.
- Fragrances: about 14 different chemicals that are hormone disruptors.
- Oxybenzone: Sunscreen agent that disrupts the hormone system.
- Parabens: these are estrogen mimicking chemicals that have been found in 19 out of 20 Breast Cancer tumors.
- PEG: probable human carcinogen.
- Phthalates: carcinogenic.
- Triclosan: antimicrobial in soap which disrupts thyroid and reproductive hormones.

In a review of evidence, the Department of Toxicology[145] in Yorkshire, UK, concluded that estrogenic chemicals through the application of body care products are adversely affecting human health. ***Parabens have been found to be estrogenic and have been found in human breast tissue.***

ANTI-PERSPIRANTS AND DEODORANTS

Believe it or not, your body was designed to sweat. Sweating is a normal and natural function that rids your body of toxins. Applying anti-perspirants clogs the pores in the arm pit with aluminum. This area of the body is very dense with sweat glands and lymph nodes in order to drain the toxins *away* from the breast. Aluminum levels are significantly higher[146] in the breast tissue of women who have Breast Cancer. **Aluminum acts like a metallo-estrogen that can mimic estrogen[147] in the breast tissue**.

---

[145] http://thermologyonline.org/Research/Breast/EndocrineDisruptersBCA.pdf
[146] http://www.ncbi.nlm.nih.gov/pubmed/21337589
[147] http://onlinelibrary.wiley.com/doi/10.1002/jat.1135/abstract

COSMETICS

This would include everything from makeup to add color to your face and lips to polishes you use on your nail beds. More than 500 products that are sold in the U.S. contain ingredients that are banned in the European Union, Canada, and Japan. Sixty-one percent of lipsticks contain residues of lead. Many of the chemicals used in cosmetics are hormone disruptors and potentially carcinogenic.[148]

Did you realize that your nails are porous and need to breathe? That means that anything that you put on your nails inevitably ends up in your body. The chemicals in nail polish, such as phthalates and formaldehyde, are classified as possible carcinogens and are hormone disruptors. Need I say more?

The good news is that there are more and more companies that are manufacturing healthy, non-toxic body care products. You can research the products on the Environmental Work Group's website. A few of my favorites are Miessence[149] and Ava Anderson Non Toxic[150].

FEMININE PROTECTION

"Make it easy to stay fresh" slogans have millions of innocent women running for the prettiest and most fragrant form of protection on the market. The average woman who lives in North America uses over 11,000 tampons or pads during her menstrual life.[151] Since you are applying these products to very sensitive skin, both externally and internally, you are subjecting your reproductive organs to an onslaught of chemicals. These feminine products contain dioxins (a byproduct of bleach) and phthalates (to make tampons glide more easily) which are carcinogenic.

---

148 http://www.ewg.org/skindeep/myths-on-cosmetics-safety/

149 http://www.miessence.com/

150 http://www.avaandersonnontoxic.com/drv

151 http://askville.amazon.com/AMERICAN-WOMEN-TAMPONS-PADS-PERIOD/AnswerViewer.do?requestId=15177503

HAIR DYES

Since I started graying when I was 19, this was a tough one for me to let go of. But in February of 2013, I took the plunge and vowed to go natural and let my silver shine through. It was a little scary at first. I felt a little vulnerable and wondered if my silver hair would age me. But I decided to 'walk my talk'. How could I tell women to reduce their toxic exposure when I was still applying that toxic dye to my head every month?

Here are a few compelling reasons to stop dyeing your hair with artificial dyes:

- Hair dyes contain chemicals that are endocrine disruptors.
- The ingredients in hair dyes are potentially carcinogenic and pose a significant health risk to those that use them and apply them. Past studies have linked hair dye to various cancers such as Breast and Ovarian.
- Lead in hair dye has been associated with harmful effects to every organ in your body.

SHAMPOOS AND SOAPS

What you put ON your skin ends up IN your body. The ingredients in regular soaps and shampoo are shocking! They are full of toxins that affect your Immune System, cause cancer, and disrupt your hormones.

The worst ingredient in soap is the antibacterial chemical called triclosan.

Triclosan was originally classified as a pesticide but somehow found its way into the household and personal care products.

Even if your soap does not say antibacterial, it can still be found in a number of soaps. It is also used in mouthwashes, toothpastes, deodorants, bedding, washcloths, and towels. Triclosan has been implicated in allergies and the growth of some cancers.[152]

Mark David created a fabulous web site about the toxins in your everyday shampoos.[153] He lost his mother to cancer when he was 12 years old. He has since been on a quest to educate and inform the world about healthier and safer choices.

TOOTHPASTE

If you read the back of a typical commercial toothpaste tube you will see a warning: *Harmful if swallowed. Call poison control center if swallowed.* Now I don't know about you but putting something in my mouth that is poisonous if swallowed does not sound like a good idea. Even if you do not physically swallow it, you are 'eating' the chemicals anyway. The lining of your mouth and the skin under your tongue are extremely rich in capillaries.

If someone is prescribed nitroglycerin for potential heart attacks, they are told to put it under their tongue. Why? ***Because anything that you put under your tongue by-passes digestion and goes directly into the blood stream.***

Therefore, if you have a mouthful of toxic toothpaste, you are ingesting those chemicals several times per day. Here is a list of some of the chemicals you should be concerned about:

- SLS or sodium lauryl sulphate – classified as a pesticide by the EPA because it is used as a flea and tick shampoo for dogs and cats. It acts as a foaming agent and is carcinogenic.
- Fluoride – a whole book could be written on the serious effects of fluoride. Exposure to fluoride can lead to bone fractures in adults and bone cancer in boys. It lowers the IQ of children and cause distortions in brain cells. It is classified as a hormone disruptor by the National Research Council and has shown

---

[152] http://www.foxnews.com/health/2012/08/14/chemical-in-many-antibacterial-soaps-linked-with-impaired-muscle-function/

[153] http://www.endalldisease.com/poison-shampoo-the-shockingly-toxic-ingredients-in-your-shampoo-exposed/

significant effects on the thyroid and parathyroid. It calcifies the pineal gland, which is associated with lower melatonin production.

- Triclosan – an antibacterial chemical found in soaps.
- Sodium Saccharin – Artificial sweetener that causes cancer.
- Artificial colors and flavorings - most of them are carcinogenic and neurotoxic.

Here is a simple check list you can use to start reducing your toxic exposure in your body. Simply check off the box when you have eliminated one of the products. You will see yourself making progress before you know it. Even 1 check mark is a great step in the right direction.

Lotions and Potions

- Face wash
- Shaving cream
- Facial moisturizers
- Anti-perspirants
- Body soaps and washes
- Sunscreens
- Body moisturizers
- Anti-bacterial hand soaps

Cosmetics

- Foundation
- Lip Gloss
- Lipstick
- Blush
- Eye shadow
- Eye liner
- Mascara

Feminine Protection

Hair Products

- Shampoo
- Conditioner
- Hair dye
- Hair sprays and gels

Dental Products

- Toothpaste
- Mouthwash

INTERNAL TOXINS

Internal toxins are what you will find inside the body that can increase your toxic load. Waste byproducts can be produced from every day metabolism and digestion of foods. If the detoxification pathways are stagnant and not functioning properly, toxins can accumulate in your body. The increased toxic load will affect your health on a cellular level and impede your body's natural healing ability.

THE COLON

Most people shy away from talking about bowel movements and habits in the bathroom, but the reality is that a constipated and clogged colon can increase your risk for Breast Cancer.

The large intestine is responsible for absorption of water and excretion of waste material. If the waste material is not properly excreted on a daily basis, the toxins will recirculate throughout the body. This toxic build up can cause cellular stress, weaken the Immune System, and increase the overall acidity in your body, which cancer cells love.[154]

---

154 http://www.ncbi.nlm.nih.gov/pubmed/22738122

Mr. V.E Irons, well known for his colon cleansing programs[155], spent years researching and advocating the need to detox the bowels in order to prevent any 'disease' in the body.

He identified 22 toxic chemicals that were produced as a result of a toxic colon and then reabsorbed into the body.

- Ammonia, phenols, indoles, and amines which have been shown to exert toxic effects in vitro and in animal models.
- Methylguanidine, a poisonous by product of protein putrefaction.
- Sepsin, a poison formed from the putrefaction of protein matter.

A simple and inexpensive way to cleanse your colon and your liver is by incorporating coffee enemas in your healing journey. There is evidence that the great Pharaohs of Egypt had a special doctor or 'guardian of the anus' that specialized in administering the enemas. In the early 1900s, German scientists noticed that caffeine opened the bile ducts and stimulated the liver of laboratory animals when coffee enemas were administered. Believe it or not, coffee enemas were in the medical Doctor's 'Bible', *The Merk Manual* until 1972.

There are certain phyto nutrients in the coffee that stimulate glutathione production on the cells. Glutathione is a primary and powerful anti-oxidant. There are various types of enema kits on the Internet. Make sure you use a stainless steel container with silicone tubing. This is the one I personally use and recommend.[156]

Regular colonic irrigations are extremely beneficial. I have used a home colonic irrigation system with the colema board[157] since the early 1980s. It is simple, private, inexpensive, and lasts forever.

To improve your elimination on a daily basis, I suggest you purchase a small stepping stool to place at the base of the toilet. I have practiced this since the 1970s when I discovered how toilets have ruined the

---

[155] http://www.veirons.com/
[156] http://breastcancerconqueror.com/store/products/coffee-enema-kit/
[157] http://www.colema.com/

colons of humans for centuries. If you watch any animal eliminate, they get into a squatting position in order to open up the pelvic muscles for proper elimination. We are no different.

Our body is designed to prevent evacuation when we are sitting or standing. When we sit, the rectum is tightened by the pubo-rectal muscles, which is designed to keep the poop in. Squatting, on the other hand, releases the muscle and allows for evacuation without straining or pushing. There are various types of stools that can be purchased but my all-time favorite is the Squatty Potty.[158] They have plain plastic models as well as beautifully designed bamboo models. If you are serious about colon cleansing, proper elimination is a great first step.

THE LIVER

The liver has over 500 various functions, one of the key functions being detoxification. It can become sluggish and toxic as a result of eating processed foods, alcohol consumption, and certain drugs and pharmaceuticals. Just like the colon, if the liver is not properly cleansed, toxins will re-circulate and cause a systemic overload. There are numerous herbs to help cleanse and detoxify the liver.

KIDNEYS

Every day, your kidneys filter about 200 quarts of blood to remove excess water and waste products. If they become clogged with uric acid crystals and other toxins, your blood will become impure and full of toxins.

PARASITES

The thought of parasites crawling inside of us is very disgusting. An excellent book you must read to bring the reality of problems with parasites is *Guess What Came to Dinner*[159], by Anne Louise Gittleman.

---

[158] http://www.squattypotty.com/?Click=24574

[159] http://www.amazon.com/Guess-What-Came-Dinner-Parasites/dp/1583330968

International travel, the food industry, and poor sanitary habits have created a parasitic epidemic.

If you have never done a parasite cleanse, chances are you are loaded with them. Parasites are a toxic burden and stress the Immune System, but their waste matter can also leave your body feeling tired and toxic. How do we get infected with parasites?

- From unclean food sources and the many hands that touch your food from the field to the grocery store.
- From other people who have poor sanitary habits.
- We can inhale the eggs, especially if we have pets.
- We come into contact with the parasites through our skin, especially the bottom of our feet.

CHRONIC INFECTIONS

According to IARC (International Agency for Research on Cancer, an intergovernmental agency associated with the WHO), one of the main causes of cancer are chronic infections, viral, bacterial, or parasitic.[160] The mechanism for causing cancer may be direct by producing oncogenic proteins, or indirectly, by creating chronic inflammation and burdening the Immune System.

When I was in active practice and tested patients with a Bio-Energetic Meridian testing device, it was very common to find low grade, chronic bacterial, viral, and fungal infections that were weakening the Immune System.

Dr. Tulio Simoncini, oncologist and cancer researcher, wrote a fascinating book called *Cancer is Fungus*.[161] His research and 20 years of success with various types of cancer has shown that at the base of neoplastic formations (tumors) there are fungal colonies. The co-existence of Candida and cancer have been seen anywhere from 79% to 97% in the tissues of cancer patients, especially in the terminally ill ones. His personal experience with thousands of cancer patients has

---

160 http://www.iarc.fr/en/publications/pdfs-online/wcr/2003/wcr-2.pdf
161 http://www.curenaturalicancro.com/

shown that the aggression of Candida causes tumors and the spread of the cancer.

Amazingly, his cure for various types of cancer is Sodium Bicarbonate. Since cancer thrives in an acidic environment and the external pH of solid tumors is acidic, then he simply blasts the cancer with a very alkaline and safe substance, baking soda.

A study of mouse models with metastatic Breast Cancer using oral sodium bicarbonate increased the pH of the tumors and reduced the spread of cancer.[162]

Sodium Bicarbonate can be used intravenously, orally, rectally, vaginally, and even local perfusions and injections of superficial and local tumors such as Breast Cancers.

I personally consulted with a woman in Europe who was treated by Dr. Simoncini. Her breast tumor had reached the point that it was too large to be reduced with simply an internal protocol. The tumor load had to be reduced either through surgery or injected with Baking Soda. She chose Dr. Simoncini's method and achieved great success. Mission accomplished! Tumor gone and health restored.

In spite of his amazing results and thousands of lives that were saved, Dr. Simoncini had his medical license revoked by the Italian government and the medical establishment. They would rather torture patients with toxic chemicals and radiation that have less than a 2% chance of survival rate, than allow a doctor to use something as simple and non-toxic as baking soda. Remember that you can't patent baking soda, so there is no big cash cow at the end of that rainbow.

Here is a simple check list you can use to start reducing your internal toxic exposure. Take your time and don't try to do too much at once. I have had both professional and personal experiences with all of these cleanses. There are many companies that offer various cleansing packages. I have used Dr. Hulda Clark's products[163] because of their

---

[162] http://www.ncbi.nlm.nih.gov/pubmed/19276390

[163] http://store.yahoo.com/cgi-bin/clink?drclarkstore+kVNu4g+index.html+fdoappa100

purity and reasonable price point. Consult with your health care provider if you have any questions about any of the cleanses.

- Colon Cleanse
- Herbal Colon Cleanse
- Coffee enemas
- Green Tea enemas
- Colonics
- Squatty Potty
- Liver Cleanse
- Herbal Cleanse
- Gall Bladder Cleanse
- Parasite Cleanse
- Kidney Cleanse
- Candida Cleanse

A great web site and resource to refer to is Dr. Judy Seger's website, Complete Cleanse System[164], which focuses on how to detox and cleanse the whole body from every disease. A Naturopath for over 35 years, Dr. Judy has worked with thousands of patients, offering various and successful detox protocols.

Here are a few other guidelines for improving your detoxification experience:

- Make sure that you are drinking clean, purified water. A simple rule is to drink half your weight in ounces. If you weigh 140 pounds, then you would drink 70 ounces per day.
- Start your morning off with 1 organic squeezed lemon into a glass of water. Add 1 teaspoon baking soda to alkalize the body.

---

[164] http://completecleansesystem.com/

- Dry Skin Brushing with a loofa sponge stimulates the largest organ of your body- your skin. It also stimulates the lymphatic system to move the impurities into the blood.
- Castor Oil Packs have been used for hundreds of years as a cleansing therapy. Flannel or cotton materials are soaked in castor oil and applied over the abdomen or over the liver area specifically. A heating pad or hot water bottle is then placed over the pack for about 1 hour. Castor oil contains an extremely high amount of an unusual fatty acid called ricinoleic acid which has anti-inflammatory, anti-microbial, and pain-killing properties. Placing the castor oil packs over the abdomen helps to open up the colon and the liver for improved toxic elimination.
- Sweating is by far one of the simplest ways to detox. New research has revealed that sweating helps to eliminate heavy metals and petrochemicals that have infiltrated our environment and ultimately our body. A ground breaking study revealed that certain toxic elements were preferentially excreted through sweat rather than urine. A review of various scientific studies and literature concluded that sweating led to detoxification of heavy metals such as mercury, cadmium, lead, and arsenic.
- Hyperthermia is an excellent way to increase your Natural Killer cells, stimulate the lymph nodes, and weaken cancer cells. I love my BioMat. It lowers the cortisol levels and showers my body with alkalizing negative ions. More on that later.
- Raising your body temperature through hot detox clay or Epsom Salts baths, sun bathing, or infra-red saunas will stimulate your blood and lymph circulation, improving the detoxification process.
- Fasting is an age old physical and spiritual healing practice. There are numerous types of fasts that you can choose from, depending on your state of health. I would not recommend an extended 10 day fast if you are on a healing journey. Instead, try a 1 or 2 day fast of all raw juices or simple lemon water. Fasting allows your body to focus on healing and repairing,

rather than using up energy to digest your food. In animal studies, the only experimental approach that consistently improves survival with cancer is 'under nutrition without malnutrition.'[165]

POINTS TO PONDER

- There are clear environmental links to Breast Cancer.
- Xeno-estrogens or false estrogens increase your risk of developing Breast Cancer.
- Environmental radiation from cell phones, cell towers, and WIFI clearly cause biological damage to the body.
- The Dirty Dozen should be avoided because of the many pesticide residues, which are potent Xeno-estrogens.
- Most of the conventional household products are very carcinogenic.
- Nonstick cookware and aluminum pans are very toxic and are hormone disruptors.
- Any body-care products that you put on your skin are absorbed into your bloodstream.
- The average person is exposed to over 126 foreign chemicals every day through their body care products.
- Women who have Breast Cancer have significantly higher levels of aluminum and parabens in their breast tissue because of the daily use of anti-perspirants.
- Sixty-one percent of commercial lipsticks contain lead.
- Hair dyes contain chemicals that are carcinogenic.
- Commercial toothpastes contain Triclosan and other cancer causing agents.
- There are over 22 toxic chemicals that are produced in a sluggish and constipated colon.
- Coffee enemas were once a part of mainstream medicine.

---

165 http://www.cmaj.ca/content/early/2013/03/25/cmaj.109-4437

- Sitting on a toilet without the proper position is the #1 cause of hemorrhoids and poor elimination.
- Chronic, low grade infections can be classified as cancer triggers.
- Candida is always associated with the presence of cancer. Sodium bicarbonate is a viable alkalizing agent that destroys cancer cells.
- Detoxing the body and organs of elimination is extremely important for a successful recovery.

YOUR HEALING JOURNEY ACTION STEPS

- Become familiar with the Environmental Working Group website to learn more about your toxic exposure.
- Practice safe cell phone use by keeping it away from your body when not in use. Use the speaker phone rather than putting it close to your head.

➢ Check your bedroom and make sure there are no electronic devices in your bedroom.

➢ Unplug your WIFI at night if it is near your bedroom.

➢ Learn more about technology that reduces the effect of EMFs on your body.

➢ Try to eat only organic produce and clean, local meats.

➢ STOP using your microwave.

➢ Slowly replace your plastic containers with glass ones.

➢ Conduct a household walk through and make a note of all the products that have dangerous chemicals in them. This is the first step in creating awareness for yourself and your family.

➢ Ask your lawn company to start using bio-degradable and non-toxic fertilizers.

➢ Ask your pesticide company to provide you with a non-toxic product substitute or simply make your own.

➢ Replace 'scented' candles with non-toxic candles.

➢ Replace your 'air freshener' with essential oils.

- Throw out and recycle your nonstick and aluminum pots and pans.
- Slowly replace your CFL light bulbs with full spectrum light bulbs.
- Start substituting commercial body care products with organic and nontoxic products. You can use coconut oil as a body moisturizer.
- Stop using antiperspirants. Replace with a non-toxic version.
- Replace your hair care products with a non-toxic version.
- Be bold and show your true colors! Stop applying toxic hair dyes to your head.
- Get rid of the toxic toothpaste and purchase healthier brands.
- Plan out time for a colon cleanse.
- Become familiar with coffee or green tea enemas.
- Purchase a small stool or a Squatty Potty for improved elimination.
- Plan out time for a liver-gallbladder flush.
- Commit to drinking at least 64 ounces of clean water every day.
- Plan out time for a parasite cleanse.
- Start your day off with the juice from 1 lemon and 1 tsp. baking soda in a glass of clean water.
- Make it a point to really sweat for 30-60 minutes, at least 3 times per week.
- Plan for a 1 or 2 day fast once per week.

CHAPTER 4

ESSENTIAL #3
BALANCE YOUR ENERGY

"No problem can be solved from the same level of consciousness that created it."

~

Albert Einstein

EVERYTHING IS ENERGY

Although this concept of energy may be new to many, the idea that we are energetic beings has been established as a scientific fact for many years. According to Dr. Carlos Rubbia, Nobel Prize Laureate, we are 1 billionth physical matter and the rest is all energy. In other words, if we were to break down the physical and energetic aspects of our body, only 1 billionth of it is physical matter and the rest exists in the form of energy and light.

Our body runs on an energetic and electrical system that can be measured with instrumentation. An EEG measures electrical activity of the brain, while an EKG measures the electrical activity of the heart. Bio-energetic Meridian Testing measures electrical resistance at various acupuncture points on the hands and the feet.

Our body also emits UPEs or Ultraweak Photon Emissions.[166] The biophotons are particles of light that are part of the visible electromagnetic spectrum and are detectable only with ultra-sensitive instrumentation. We emit fewer photons in the morning and more in the evening, while our head seems to emit the most and increasingly so over the day.[167] Our DNA seems to be a type of laser that emits coherent light and communicates to our cells.[168] Scientists have recognized that the biophoton emissions become less intense when there is biochemical or biophysical stress.

Kirlian Photography is a technique that measures the electrical discharge from any living entity, human, animal, and plant. You can actually see the 'energy' in the form of a corona being emitted around the circumference of the photographed object. (Interestingly, canned foods, cooked meats, and pasteurized milk are lifeless and do not produce an electrical emission.)

What does all of this have to do with healing and preventing Breast Cancer? If we are energetic beings, then we must make sure that our energy flow is not being obstructed or impeded.

We must do everything possible to keep our energetic system strong and full of vitality.

Let's compare our body to a car battery. If the battery is low, you can't even turn on the ignition and operate the vehicle. In a similar vein, if the energetic flow of the body is low, then optimal healing cannot happen.

In this chapter, I will discuss:

- Various healing arts and how they can improve your energetic body.
- The key hormones that must be kept in balance and how to monitor them properly.
- The importance of sleep in your healing process.

---

[166] http://www.greenmedinfo.com/affiliate/2929/node/102238
[167] http://www.ncbi.nlm.nih.gov/pubmed/15947468
[168] http://www.ncbi.nlm.nih.gov/pubmed/6204761

- The necessity of exercise on a healing journey.
- Various therapies that may help balance your energetic body.

THE POWER OF CHIROPRACTIC

Before you flip to the next page or jump over this topic, I ask you to keep an open mind about this amazing profession. Simply put, your Nerve System commands and controls every single aspect of your body. It could be said that it is the Master Computer System of the body. The vertebra and your skull protect this electrical system from harm but when the vertebrae misalign or become subluxated because of physical, chemical, or emotional stress, the electrical flow of the nerve system can be impeded. Chiropractors specialize in gently realigning the spine in order to allow the brain to communicate freely with all parts of the body.

Here are a few interesting facts about your Nerve System and your Immune System:

- Immune function[169] is regulated in part by the Sympathetic Nerve System. These nerves affect the lymph nodes, the spleen, and the thymus.
- Dr. Ronald Pero, Chief of Cancer Prevention Research[170] at New York's Preventative Medicine Institute, measured the function of the Immune System of patients under Chiropractic Care versus those of the general population. ***He found on average that those under Chiropractic Care had a 300% greater Immune competence than those who had not received Chiropractic Care.*** "When applied in a clinical framework, I have never seen any group to experience such an increase. That is why it (Chiropractic) is so dramatically important."

---

169 Murray DR, Irwin M, Reardon CA, et al. "Sympathetic and immune interactions during dynamic exercise. Mediation via a beta 2 - adrenergic-dependent mechanism." Circulation 1992 86(1): 203

170 Pero R. "Medical Researcher Excited By CBSRF Project Results." The Chiropractic Journal, August 1989; 32

- The activity of specific cells of the Immune System that attack and destroy unhealthy cells is enhanced[171] through Chiropractic Care.
- Over a 6 month period, the Immune System of HIV patient[172] was enhanced by 48% compared to those that were not under Chiropractic Care.
- Dr. Felton and his researchers found that various stimuli that affect the Central Nerve System can profoundly alter the immune response[173].

I have personally been under Chiropractic Care since I was 16 years old. It changed my life forever by clearing my migraines, chronic constipation, and severe menstrual cramps. I personally have witnessed the transformation of over 18,000 patients in the course of my career, so I believe I can speak from experience when I ask you to consider incorporating Chiropractic on your healing journey. The advanced and scientific techniques that many modern day Chiropractors use are painless and very gentle.

A very proactive and well balanced group that represents the Chiropractic profession is called Maximized Living[174]. Their motto is "True health is more than just feeling good." They have created a simple system of living that will help you live a natural and healthy life. I have lectured with Maximized Living Doctors and have cousins and nephews that are a part of this group, so I can personally vouch for their passion and their mission. To find a Maximized Living Doctor[175] in your area, please visit their website.

Here are several other Healing Arts that you can benefit from while you are on your healing journey:

Acupuncture is a component of Traditional Chinese Medicine that involves stimulating specific points in order to correct the flow of

---

171 http://www.chiro.org/research/ABSTRACTS/Immune_Responses_to_Spinal_Manipulation.shtml

172 http://www.chiro.org/research/ABSTRACTS/Immune.shtml

173 http://www.ncbi.nlm.nih.gov/pmc/articles/PMC284388/

174 http://www.maximizedliving.com/

175 http://www.maximizedliving.com/Home/FindaDoctor.aspx

energy in the body. Imagine your meridians like a freeway system that gets bogged down during rush hour. The energy accumulates in certain areas of the body, creating blockages and imbalanced energy flow. The electricity that runs along the meridian system is its own separate system and integrates all the organs and teeth into one system.

As I will discuss in Chapter 6, Essential #5, Embrace Biological Dentistry, your teeth are connected to your organs through the acupuncture meridian system. A root canal or large amalgam in a tooth that corresponds to the breast can weaken the flow of energy to that area of the body, making it more susceptible to disease.

There are several professional organizations that can help you find a Diplomat of Oriental Medicine[176].

Neuromuscular Therapy or Massage is the manipulation of muscles and connective tissue to improve function and enhance the healing process. The act of 'kneading' the body releases trigger points in the muscles and helps to improve lymphatic flow. Massage is not only beneficial for you physically but it also helps to calm the soul.

A pilot study on the effectiveness of massage[177] for postsurgical mastectomies patients reported a significant reduction in pain, stress, and muscle tension, as well as an increased sense of relaxation.

If you are on a Breast Cancer healing journey, consult with your therapist about any contraindications for your massage.

Reflexology is another hands-on therapy that you may consider. The nerve endings in the feet are connected to all the organs in the body. Various locations on the soles of the feet correspond to specific organs. Applying pressure to these points can indirectly stimulate the organs. A study conducted by researchers at Michigan State

---

176 http://www.nccaom.org/

177 http://www.ncbi.nlm.nih.gov/pubmed/22459520

University found that reflexology[178] helped women in late stage Breast Cancer to have an improved quality of life.

PEMF OR PULSED ELECTROMAGNETIC FIELDS

We are well aware that there are specific elements that are required for an optimal life, but there is another element that the majority of people are not aware of, and that is PEMF. The earth emits specific frequencies and resonances that are vital for human health. They are so essential that the U.S. and Russian space programs equip their space crafts with devices that emit these frequencies.

These frequencies emitted by planet earth are necessary to maintain health and energy production. Because of toxic environmental issues, indoor living, and many hours spent working in a building, we are no longer getting this life nurturing energy from our planet. There is compelling evidence that the earth's magnetism is essential for life. In fact, research has shown that PEMF has a cytotoxic effect on Breast Cancer cells but were not damaging to healthy cells[179].

Bryant Meyers, BS, MA in Physics has written a brilliant book called *PEMF, The 5th Element*[180]. He has spent years researching PEMF therapy, which he feels is the crown jewel of energy medicine.

SOUND THERAPY

Music and sounds created with gongs, tuning forks, or Tibetan bowls are various forms of sound frequencies that have healing properties. Since everything in the Universe vibrates at various frequencies, including healthy cells and cancer cells, listening to or exposing your body to various healing sounds could have a potentially healing effect. Studies have shown that musical sounds altered the functionality and

---

178 http://www.medicalnewstoday.com/releases/31689.php
179 http://www.ncbi.nlm.nih.gov/pubmed/24039828
180 http://www.imrs2000.com/pemf-book/#.UxDb_PldV0w

shape of Breast Cancer cells as well as interfered with the hormone binding properties[181].

Since 1991, Dr. Mitchell Gaynor, M.D., Director of Medical Oncology and Integrative Medicine at the Strang-Cornell Cancer Prevention Center in New York, has used healing sounds with his patients. In his words[182]:

> ***"Sound affects us on a physiological level. Sound can change our immune function. After chanting or listening to Gregorian chants or classical music, an index in your immune system goes up between 12.5% to 15%. About 20 minutes after listening to meditative music, your immunoglobulin levels in your blood are significantly increased. There is no part of your body that is not affected."***

He has written a fascinating book called *The Healing Power of Sound*[183]. In his book, he describes how chanting, listening to music, wind gongs, hand drums, etc. can positively affect our minds as well as our bodies. All of these sounds are united by certain principles, the most important of which is the tendency toward harmony in nature.

That is a powerful message! Since most human beings spend 90% of their time inside, in a house, in a car, or in an office building, we have become so alienated from nature, its sounds, and the energetic frequencies of the earth and sun. Taking the time to relax and enjoy the sounds of music and the sounds of nature, may give you an added edge on healing your body.

LIGHT THERAPY

The technical term for light therapy is Photodynamic Therapy or PDT[184]. Patients are injected with a non-toxic photosensitizing dye that is absorbed by all cells and stays in the cancer cells much longer. When that photosensitive chemical is exposed to a specific

---

181 http://www.ncbi.nlm.nih.gov/pubmed/23955127
182 http://gongsoundhealing.com/sound-therapy/cancer-sound-healing/
183 http://amzn.com/1570629552
184 http://www.cancer.gov/cancertopics/factsheet/Therapy/photodynamic

wavelength of light, the agent produces a form of oxygen that kills cancer cells and not healthy cells. PDT appears to shrink or destroy tumors, damages the blood vessels that feed the tumor, and seems to activate the Immune System[185].

SONO-PHOTO DYNAMIC THERAPY (SPDT)

SPDT is a combination of light therapy and sound therapy that has been used successfully at the Hope 4 Cancer Institute[186] in Mexico, minutes from the San Diego, USA border. It is very similar to PDT, but the agent that is ingested sublingually is also activated by sound frequencies. The sound therapy could do best with deeper tumors because the body transmits sounds better than light.

This system is registered and allowed in 25 countries in the European Union[187]. There are approximately 3000 published research articles about this therapy.

COLOR THERAPY OR CHROMOTHERAPY

Einstein with his renowned equation of $E = mc^2$ determined that energy and physical matter are the dual expression of the same universal substance. The rate of vibration determines the density and its expression in material form. Light is electromagnetic radiation or simply a form of energy. Each color has a different frequency of vibration and thus affects the cells in various ways. Chromotherapy or light therapy is a centuries-old concept that has been used successfully to heal various diseases[188].

Many scientists believe that various colors of light entering through the eye are responsible for the biological rhythms in the body. Interestingly, even blind people are able to be affected by light and have learned to 'read' light through their fingertips. In fact, studies

---

185 http://www.nih.gov/researchmatters/december2011/12052011light.htm
186 http://www.sonophotodynamictherapy.com/index.html
187 http://www.sonophotodynamictherapy.com/sonophotodynamictherapy_therapy.html
188 http://www.ncbi.nlm.nih.gov/pmc/articles/PMC1297510/

conducted in the U.S. and Russia suggest that all living things conduct light[189].

The book *Color Medicine*[190] provides a simple technique for treating specific imbalances and strengthening the Immune System. Color Medicine utilizes subtle energy frequencies to support the healing process.

Sunlight is, of course, the perfect blend of all colors and is the ultimate form of light therapy. Since colors are responsible for the release of specific hormones which keep us healthy, exposing your body to the sun for about 1 hour per day is very beneficial.

DO YOU HAVE HAPPY HORMONES?

Hormones are included in the topic of energy since hormones are responsible for the regulation of many physiological functions and behavioral activities. Hormones are messengers that are secreted by glands and are then transported through the blood stream to target organs. They can stimulate or inhibit growth, wake you up or make you feel sleepy, can activate or suppress the Immune system, and even affect your moods.

I think we all can agree that when our hormones are out of balance, we *feel* out of balance. The discussion of balancing hormones can be a whole book unto itself, so for the sake of time and space, I will simply hit the highlights.

Unfortunately, mainstream medicine has created fear in women at the mention of their hormones. Hormones are associated with the increased risk of cancer. Billions of dollars have been banked by Big Pharma as a result of hormone suppressing drugs that are supposed to "block female hormones so the cancer won't reoccur." However, as previously discussed, the very drugs that hold promise for a cancer free future are the very ones that leave women scarred with life-long side-effects and other forms of cancer.

---

189 http://www.ncbi.nlm.nih.gov/pmc/articles/PMC1297510/
190 http://amzn.com/B00898JLS2

First and foremost for you to understand: ***YOUR hormones are not your enemy!*** Your hormones are your friend and ally. Think about this for a moment: during a woman's younger years, when sex hormones are at their highest, there are relatively fewer incidences of Breast Cancer. If **your** hormones were the sole cause of Breast Cancer, then the incidence of Breast Cancer would be much higher with this younger age group.

As you age, the cancer risk increases because of the accumulation of toxins and Xeno-estrogens, fatigue and protective genes that are turned off because of poor nutrition and poor sleep.

As you learned in the first few chapters of this book, your body is subjected to countless chemicals that stimulate estrogen production or chemically mimic estrogen in the body. The key is to reduce your exposure to these Xeno-estrogens and make sure that you are breaking down and metabolizing estrogen properly. Determine exactly what your hormone levels are with a simple home saliva test[191] so you can monitor your hormones. There are also reliable urine tests[192] that assess the risk of estrogen related diseases.

The most reliable way to determine your biologically available hormones is through Saliva Testing[193]*.* There are 2 forms of hormones in your blood: they are either connected to a protein or are 'free' hormones. The hormones connected to proteins are 'unavailable' because they are too large. The unattached or free hormones are the only hormones that are bio-available for delivery to the receptor sites in the body. The hormones that are attached to proteins are too large to fit into the receptor cites on the cells and are, therefore, useless.

Blood serum testing measures all the hormones in the blood, including those that are not bio-available. However, when blood is filtered through the salivary glands, the free hormones can pass through the filters in the saliva glands while the large, protein bound hormones cannot.

---

191 http://breastcancerconquerorshop.com/product/comprehensive-saliva-plus-panel/

192 http://breastcancerconquerorshop.com/product/estrogens-urinalysis-essential/

193 http://www.labrix.com/InformationResearch

Thus, saliva testing tells us what hormones are actually available for your body to put to use. Since hormones are powerful messenger molecules that affect our physical and mental health, balancing your hormones is an important part of your healing journey.

The first step in understanding your hormones is learning about your EQ or Estrogen Quotient[194]. The Estrogen Quotient is a formula developed by Dr. Henry Lemon that examines all 3 types of estrogens in a specific ratio.

The 3 types of estrogen are:

E1 or Estrone is the least abundant of the estrogens and is most abundant in postmenopausal women. It can be converted to estradiol, the more aggressive estrogen.

E2 or Estradiol is 10 times more potent that Estrone and about 80 times more potent than Estriol or E3. Estradiol is the predominant estrogen during reproductive years and has been linked to the development of various female cancers such as Breast, Ovarian, and Uterine Cancer. I believe that this estrogen is the dominant form of estrogen that is introduced through various chemicals in the environment and in body care products.

E3 or Estriol is the gentler estrogen and has a protective effect against 'cellular growth factors' of the other estrogens. Estriol reduces the effect[195] of the more aggressive estradiol and has a protective effect against radiation-induced cancer of the breast[196].

When all 3 estrogens levels are known, then a mathematical formula called the EQ Ratio (Estrogen Quotient) can be applied. This formula was developed by Dr. Henry Lemon in his studies of estriol, the gentle estrogen, and how it pertained to Breast Cancer in humans. If your ratio of the more aggressive estrogens, E1 and E2, are higher than the less aggressive estrogen, E3, then your chances of developing cancer may be greater.

---

194 http://breastcancerconqueror.com/how-to-balance-hormones/
195 http://www.ncbi.nlm.nih.gov/pubmed/9369454
196 http://www.ncbi.nlm.nih.gov/pubmed/2702580

In other words, the higher the EQ, the lower your risk of Breast Cancer. Fortunately, there is no need to try to figure this out on your own as this is part of a Comprehensive Plus Hormone Panel that is readily available[197]. Order the kit, and it is delivered to your home. Follow the simple instructions and send the kit back to the lab. Within a few weeks, the ordering physician gets the results and reviews them with you.

- Another step in understanding your hormone balance is to determine if you are metabolizing estrogen properly[198]. If you are not breaking down estrogen properly because of a sluggish liver or if you have a problem with methylation, you may not be effectively eliminating carcinogenic hormone metabolites. Long term estrogen dominance is a significant risk factor in developing Breast Cancer.

Once you have gathered this information through blood work or urine tests, your health care provider can make necessary recommendations. If you are pre-menopausal, changes in your diet, herbal and nutritional support for your endocrine system, as well as detoxification can help bring your EQ ration to a healthier level.

If you are post-menopausal, bio-identical hormone supplementation may be beneficial for you. There is a tremendous amount of ignorance in the traditional medical community regarding bio-identical hormones and, therefore, you will need to find a doctor that understands the need for bio-identical hormone therapy.

Bio-identical hormones share the exact same molecular structure as those that we produce in our body. They are typically applied as a cream or gel on the surface of the skin. Dr. Jonathan Wright, M.D. recommends that topical bio-identical creams be formulated as a 'tri-estrogen formula'[199]. This replicates the ratio of estrogens that are normally found in the body.

---

[197] http://breastcancerconqueror.com/store/products/comprehensive-plus-panel/
[198] http://breastcancerconqueror.com/store/products/complete-hormones-urinalysis/
[199] http://www.tahomaclinic.com/

The ratio is as follows:

90% Estriol, 7% Estradiol, 3% Estrone

Other schools of thought suggest that estriol can be used alone, since it such a protective and gentle estrogen. Still others recommend 50% estriol and 50% estradiol in a compounded formula.

Additional hormones such as progesterone, testosterone, and DHEA may be added to the formulation, depending on the results of the saliva tests.

The big question that often comes up is, "Are bio-identical hormones safe to take if I have Breast Cancer?" The answer is yes.

A large study following tens of thousands of women conducted by Dr. Agnes Fournier found there was no increase in Breast Cancer-related to bio-identical hormone therapy[200]. In fact, women who were using bio-identical hormones had a 10% decrease in the risk of Breast Cancer.

The European Menopause Journal[201] published an article about the difference between synthetic and bio-identical hormones. This was their conclusion: "Compelling indications also exist that differences might also be present for the risk of developing breast cancer, with recent trials indicating that the association of natural progesterone with estrogens *confers less or even no risk of breast cancer* as opposed to the use of other synthetic progestins."

If you choose to use bio-identical hormones or if your EQ ratio is out of balance, consider supplementing with DIM and I3C[202], which is a concentration of compounds found in cruciferous vegetables that help to metabolize and process harmful estrogen metabolites.

As stated in my disclaimer, I am not a medical doctor, and I am not giving you medical advice. Consult with a physician that is supportive

---

200 http://www.virginiahopkinstestkits.com/bioidenticalbreastcancer.html

201 http://www.maturitas.org/article/S0378-5122%2808%2900204-1/abstract

202 http://breastcancerconquerorshop.com/product/dim-i3c-healthy-estrogen-support/

of Bio-identical hormones and understands how to prescribe them properly.

THE SLEEP-CANCER CONNECTION

Healthy restful sleep is an essential part of keeping your body in balance.

According to Dr. Stan Burzynski, an internationally known physician and cancer specialist,

"Stress and lack of sleep can silence cancer-protective genes."

Restful, refreshing, and rejuvenating sleep is orgasmic. There is nothing like waking up in the morning after 7-8 hours of sleep, ready to take on the day. On the flipside, if you have not had enough sleep, if you have tossed and turned and have watched the hours go by, you are dreading the day and what lies ahead. I can speak from personal experience on this matter.

As a child I remember my mother complaining of having another 'nuit blanche', which translated from French means a 'white night' or no sleep. I could not relate to that at all until I turned 40. The change of hormones and very stressful events brought on many of those 'white nights'. For years, I struggled with insomnia and those dreaded mornings I had to face after only a few hours of sleep.

I spent years researching sleep and all the hormones and neurotransmitters involved in the sleep pattern. In my research, I came across saliva and urine neurotransmitter sleep panels that analyzed the various neurotransmitters and hormones such as serotonin, GABA, dopamine, epinephrine, norepinephrine, and glutamate. My results were off the charts! No wonder I could not sleep.

With proper supplementation of L-theanine, Glutamate, tryptophan, and other supportive herbs, I can proudly say that 9:10 times, I sleep a solid 7 - 8 hours and sleep like a baby! I wake up refreshed and revitalized and ready to take on the day. I LOVE that feeling, and I am so grateful for it because I know what it is like to really suffer (and it is suffering) from insomnia.

I am so thankful and blessed to have discovered the key to a good night's sleep. If you would like more information about the sleep profile that changed my life and the lives of countless other people, visit this link on my web site[203].

Now back to the importance of sleep.

Sleep is an active process and a time when your body detoxifies, heals, and regenerates. Physiological changes occur in brain activity, heart rate, blood pressure, respiration, and temperature, depending on the stage of sleep. Many hormones are released during sleep, one of them being the Growth Hormone, which is related in part to repairing the body.

As human beings, our bodies are endowed with a biological clock or a circadian rhythm. This biological process runs on 24 hour cycles and is associated with sunlight and darkness. Emerging data is showing us how important it is to stay in sync with our biological clocks. In fact, stress related disruptions in our patterns, such as insufficient sleep, may affect a cancer prognosis[204].

Disrupted sleep patterns can induce cancer progression and growth.

Poor sleep patterns promote insulin resistance and a decrease in the satiety hormone leptin, a hormone that signals appetite control[205]. High insulin levels and obesity have been clearly linked to cancer. Sleep loss also affects the thyroid, which leads to weight gain, perpetuating the vicious cycle[206].

---

203 http://breastcancerconquerorshop.com/product/neuro-hormone-complete-panel/
204 http://www.ncbi.nlm.nih.gov/pubmed/12946654?dopt=Abstract
205 http://www.ncbi.nlm.nih.gov/pubmed/20042408
206 http://www.medscape.org/viewarticle/502825

But most importantly, your Immune System is affected by your sleep patterns. Research has shown us that people who had difficultly going to sleep had lower levels of Natural Killer Cells[207].

Incandescent light bulbs and our electronic devices such as television, computers, book pads, and I pads, have disrupted our circadian patterns. When light enters your eyes, it affects a small gland in your brain called the hypothalamus, also known as 'the brain's brain'. This gland controls blood pressure, body temperature, thirst reflex, hunger, stress response, emotions, and the Immune System. That's a powerful little gland!

If the hypothalamus is not receiving full spectrum sunlight, our biological rhythms are disrupted. Ideally, we should have at least 1 hour of sunlight shining in our eyes every day. Unfortunately, the office buildings and most homes are delivering fluorescent lights and incomplete light.

Since the hypothalamus is also connected to the pineal gland that secretes Melatonin, the sleep/wake cycle is affected. ***Melatonin is not only a 'sleep' hormone, but it is also categorized as a cytotoxic hormone which acts as a scavenger attacking free radicals.*** Having sufficient levels of melatonin is very important to prevent cancer as well as to heal from cancer[208].

- Melatonin suppresses Breast Cancer cell growth.
- Dr. David Blask, M.D., Ph.D., a cancer biology expert, conducted several experiments that proved that melatonin slowed Breast Cancer cell growth by 70%[209].
- Melatonin counteracts the effect of excess estrogen and the effect estrogen has on Breast Cancer cells.
- Melatonin reduces oxidative stress in the body.
- Melatonin reduces the side effects from chemotherapy and radiation.

---

207 http://www.psychosomaticmedicine.org/content/60/1/48.abstract

208 http://breastcancerconqueror.com/7-ways-melatonin-acts-as-a-breast-cancer-inhibitor/

209 http://tulane.edu/news/newwave/121108_blask.cfm

- Melatonin boosts your Immune System.
- Melatonin causes apoptosis or cancer cell death.
- High doses of Melatonin (10-50 mg) have proven beneficial in treating various types of cancers.

Since Melatonin peaks when there is total darkness, you can see how important it is to create a 'sleep sanctuary' in your bedroom. Here are a few suggestions that may improve your sleep patterns.

- Turn off all those electronic devices, including the television, by 9 p.m. Read a relaxing book or meditate to soothing music.
- Remove all electronic devices from your bedroom. That includes cell phones, iPads, computers, etc. If your WIFI router is near your bedroom, turn it off for the night. EMFs reduce the effect Melatonin has on cancer cells.
- If you must have an 'alarm' clock in your room, keep it at least 6 feet from your head. Set the wake up sound that is something relaxing and soothing. Why start your day with a stress response?
- Make sure your bedroom is totally dark. No night lights or street lights. Hang dark curtains. If this does not work, then wear an eye mask that blocks out all the light.
- Keep the temperature between 65 - 69 degrees Fahrenheit.
- Create a routine when it comes to bed time. Try to get to bed at the same time every night.
- Avoid alcohol and caffeine before bed time.

If you are having challenges with sleep, I encourage you to have your neurotransmitters tested to see what hormones are out of balance[210].

Sleep is a natural body function that can be restored. Something has happened along the way to affect and interrupt your sleep patterns.

---

[210] http://breastcancerconquerorshop.com/product/neuro-hormone-complete-panel/

Please, do NOT fall into the temptation of a quick fix with sleeping pills. These do NOT address the cause of your insomnia and do not provide the real, restful sleep that your body needs.

According to Dr. Daniel F. Kripke, M.D., people who take sleeping pills die sooner than people who do not use sleeping pills[211]. In a study of over 10,000 people who took sleeping pills, those who averaged 132 pills per year died 4.6 times as often as those who did not take sleeping pills and were ***35% more likely to develop a new cancer***.

DO I HAVE TO EXERCISE?

The simple answer is yes. ☺

Don't throw your hands up in the air and think, "How can I exercise when I am on this healing journey?" Or, the other excuse is, "But I HATE to exercise." Exercise comes in various shapes, sizes, and forms. The action of moving your body is what is important, since that moves the blood and the lymph throughout the body. Moving your body affects and balances your energy in many ways.

According to the National Cancer Institute[212], a panel of 13 researchers have concluded that the most important message for people who want to prevent cancer or heal from cancer more effectively, is to avoid inactivity. In other words, move your body!

Do you need some proof that exercise can help prevent Breast Cancer? Hopefully, these studies can motivate you to start moving your body:

- In a year-long study, a 38% reduced risk of invasive Breast Cancer was seen in women who did heavy lifting and carrying versus sitting on their butts all day[213].
- Moderate activity after menopause can contribute to a reduction of Breast Cancer[214].

---

211 http://www.darksideofsleepingpills.com/
212 http://www.cancer.gov/ncicancerbulletin/062910/page5
213 http://www.ncbi.nlm.nih.gov/pubmed/20864719
214 http://www.ncbi.nlm.nih.gov/pubmed/20607384

- Physical exercise alters sex hormones and their receptors in a way that causes cancer cell death or apoptosis[215].
- Certain proteins that are rich in cysteine are secreted from muscle tissue during exercise[216]. These proteins slow down tumor growth by causing apoptosis or cancer cell death.
- Exercise controls insulin levels, which is very important for cancer prevention.
- Exercise improves immune function, antioxidant activity, and promotes DNA repair[217].
- According to an expert panel of the WHO, the most physically active women reduced the risk of developing Breast Cancer by 20-40%[218].

For those women that are on a healing journey with Breast Cancer, there is mounting evidence that movement and activity helps to improve survival rates and overcome the effects of traditional therapies.

In a summary provided by the Cochrane Collaboration[219], 56 studies involving over 4000 patients suggested that aerobic activity such as walking or bike riding helped to reduce fatigue in people with Breast Cancer and Prostate Cancer.

For women undergoing radiation therapy, a 6 minute walk caused a substantial decline of the side effects on the lungs and heart[220]. Imagine the improvement you could feel if you stretched that walk to 30 minutes.

---

215 http://www.ncbi.nlm.nih.gov/pubmed/22830442
216 http://www.ncbi.nlm.nih.gov/pubmed/22851666
217 http://www.bmj.com/content/321/7274/1424
218 http://jama.jamanetwork.com/article.aspx?articleid=200955#REF-JOC50040-4
219 http://summaries.cochrane.org/CD006145/the-effect-of-exercise-on-fatigue-associated-with-cancer
220 http://www.ncbi.nlm.nih.gov/pubmed/23788992

In a controlled study, women who endured high dose chemotherapy agreed to train for 6 weeks in an endurance training program[221]. These women had lower fatigue scores and higher hemoglobin levels.

According to the Macmillan Cancer Support Group, being active during and after cancer treatment can help reduce fatigue, reduce stress and anxiety, as well as strengthen your bones and heart[222].

Simply walking the equivalent of 3 to 5 hours per week which is 25 minutes to 43 minutes per day greatly reduced the risk of death from Breast Cancer[223].

Make the walking a pleasant experience. Listen to soothing or upbeat music, whatever you are in the mood for. Stretch before and after the walk. Drink plenty of water before and after.

Why not incorporate light weights in your post exercise stretch?

If walking seems boring to you, there are so many benefits from other forms of healing exercises routines such as yoga, Tai-Chi, and Chi-gong. Join a class and make it part of your daily routine. If you are not feeling well enough to travel and drive, YouTube has many free videos from which to choose.

Have you ever heard of rebounding? This involves jumping on a mini-trampoline, also known as a rebounder. Rebounding has been studied by NASA and is a recommended form of exercise. Rebounding helps to move the lymphatic fluid and has less impact on your joints than running.

If you are physically able to rev up your intensity to your exercise routine, then you can try 'burst training'. Burst training is intense activity that pushes your body for 20 minutes[224]. Studies in the *Journal of Physiology* have found that 20 minutes of high intensity training has many benefits.

---

221 http://onlinelibrary.wiley.com/doi/10.1002/1097-0142(20010915)92:6%2B%3C1689::AID-CNCR1498%3E3.0.CO;2-H/pdf

222 http://www.macmillan.org.uk/Cancerinformation/Livingwithandaftercancer/Physicalactivity/Physicalactivityandcancer/Benefits.aspx

223 http://jama.jamanetwork.com/article.aspx?articleid=200955

224 http://breastcancerconqueror.com/why-spend-1-hour-in-the-gym/

Regardless of the type of activity that you choose, make sure that you are physically able and that you inform your primary care provider.

POINTS TO PONDER

- Since your body is only 1 billionth physical matter, keeping our energetic body balanced is a key to vibrant health.
- On average, people under Chiropractic Care have a 300% greater Immune competence than those who have not received Chiropractic Care.
- Acupuncture balances the meridian and energetic flow of the body and may thus improve healing.
- Neuromuscular therapy or massage has been shown to reduce pain, stress, and muscle tension for postsurgical mastectomy patients.
- Your hormones do not cause cancer. If that were the case, every 21 year old on this planet would be ravaged with cancer.
- It is your exposure to environmental xeno-estrogens that increase your risk for Breast Cancer.
- Your ability to properly metabolize the estrogens in your body is extremely important for cancer prevention.
- Your Estrogen Quotient, or your EQ, is a simple way to assess a possible Breast Cancer risk.
- Supplementation with DIM and I3C may improve estrogen metabolism.
- Sleep is a normal and natural body function that can be restored.
- Disrupted sleep patterns can induce cancer progression and growth.
- Melatonin suppresses Breast Cancer cell growth and causes apoptosis to cancer cells.
- People using sleeping pills are 35% more likely to develop a new cancer.

- Exercise reduces your risk of developing Breast Cancer and decreases your mortality rate if you have Breast Cancer.
- Walking 25 to 43 minutes per day provides extremely beneficial results.

YOUR HEALING JOURNEY ACTION STEPS

- ➢ Consider seeing a Chiropractor such as those associated with Maximized Living.
- ➢ Include acupuncture in your healing journey.
- ➢ Schedule an appointment with a professional and licensed Massage therapist that has experience with whole body healing.
- ➢ Discover your EQ ratio (Estrogen Quotient) by having your hormones analyzed with saliva testing.
- ➢ Examine your sleep patterns. If you are not getting 7-8 hours of restful, revitalizing sleep, consider doing a Sleep Neurotransmitter Profile.
- ➢ If you are relying on sleeping pills, get professional help to break that addiction.
- ➢ Consider incorporating Melatonin in your supplementation regime.
- ➢ Commit to 25 to 43 minutes of walking every day.
- ➢ If your body is strong enough, learn about the benefits of burst training.

Chapter 5

Essential #4 – Heal Your Emotional Wounds

"Our deepest wounds surround our greatest gifts."

~

Ken Page

For some of you, this may be the most difficult chapter to read and get through. It will require you to be brutally honest with yourself and with others. I must admit that healing my emotional wounds was the most difficult part of my healing.

Being quite an analytical and logical thinker, I could relate to the facts, the science, and the biology of a healing journey. I became aware of the need to heal my emotional wounds when I was 13 and continued to see several therapists over the course of my adult life. I thought I had it all figured out....I was 'OK'.

But my experience with Breast Cancer was sending me another message: "You are not done with your emotional healing. You still have 'stuff' to let go of and heal." Emotional healing can be scary and leave you feeling very vulnerable, so I ask you to trust the process and follow the suggestions outlined in this chapter.

I speak from my heart as I write these words. I truly understand what it is like to be burdened with emotional stress and pain. My childhood was filled with stress, strife, and the damaging effects of parental alcoholism. It pains me to write those words, but my parents' own unresolved wounds hindered their parenting skills. They were wounded children themselves and, therefore, did not know how to nurture and be present for their children. I love them and have forgiven them since I now understand why they lived their lives the way they did.

With very little attention and nurturing, I was left on my own to play by myself and wander the neighborhood. Our next door neighbor, a convicted pedophile, preyed on that opportunity and inflicted physical and emotional wounds that still bring tears to my eyes when I think of 'that little girl'. I was an innocent child that just wanted to be loved and protected. Instead, I was abused and lost faith and trust in men and in humanity.

Those formative years were the basis for the development of my teen age and adult life. I matured physically but emotionally, I was a confused, scared, scarred, and a wounded child.

After hundreds of hours of therapy and countless books, I began to understand why I had sabotaged my life time and time again. Although I was very successful in my practice and a powerful business woman, subconsciously, I felt so undeserving of true, enduring, and stable love.

However, with prayer, perseverance, and my commitment to a happier life, I learned to heal and let go of the dark gloom and doom that festered inside my soul.

I was finally able to cast away my dark demons that had kept me captive my whole life.

I have felt hopeless and helpless. I have been despondent and depressed.

Fortunately, there was a seed of greatness inside of me that kept germinating and taking root as I peeled away the layers of dysfunction.

Happy became my new normal. Happy and healthy can become your new normal!

I finally was able to cast away my dark demons that had kept me captive all my life. So you see, not to sound too cliché, but true health is not a destination, it is a journey. If you are not growing and stretching, you are become stale and stagnant.

I share my personal story to let you know that I understand emotional pain. I understand suppression that leads to depression. You, too, can let go of the dark gloomy thoughts and replace them with sunny, bubbly happy thoughts.

If you *really* want to get well and heal your body, this chapter is one of the more important ones. If you skip this information and think you have it all together, you are missing a BIG piece of the puzzle. Sadly, I have seen women on a healing journey who believe they have it all together. They compartmentalize their disease and keep functioning like everything is fine and OK. They continue to do the car pooling and all the children's activities, work full time, and carry on without stopping to rest and take inventory of the more important things.

These 'super moms' and 'super women' often lose their battle with cancer because they keep putting themselves last on the list of 'things to do'.

They do not take the time to rest, meditate, and heal the emotional wounds that may have initiated the cancer in the first place.

WILL YOU BE BITTER OR BETTER?

Being diagnosed with cancer is scary and surreal. You never think it can happen to you. The initial shock and trauma of the diagnosis can leave you paralyzed for weeks and sometimes months. There is typically the initial shock, then disbelief, which often leads to "Why me?" then anger, frustration, and eventually acceptance.

You can spend your energy on being angry and complaining about being a victim of your genes and your life, or you can use that energy to visualize yourself being victorious over the cancer and being healthy, whole, and complete.

The truth is it is not so much what happens to us, but how we deal with what happens to us. You ultimately have a choice. You can be bitter or you can choose to be better.

YOU can look at this cancer as a curse or as a blessing.

Blessing? You are probably thinking I am out of my mind to suggest that cancer can be a blessing. In his book, *Getting Well Again*[225], Dr. Carl Simonton beautifully describes the message of cancer as being a message of love:

"The need to refocus is the greatest message of cancer. Over and over again, I have seen cancer as the body's way of shocking a person into making changes. I believe cancer is a message to stop doing the things that bring you pain, and start doing the things that bring you joy - things that are more in line with who you are and what you want your life to become."

In other words, if you keep doing the things you have always done, you will keep getting the same results. YOU HAVE TO CHANGE.

You have to change your emotional patterns, your communication styles, your forgiveness and tolerance, your stress management, and your pace of life. You can design and create a life that brings you laughter, playfulness, and joy.

If you have read this far, I applaud you for being brave and courageous. I promise you that if stay the course in this chapter and do the work, you will transform into a happier, healthier you.

---

[225] http://amzn.com/0553280333

DO YOU HAVE THE 'CANCER PERSONALITY'?

In Chapter 1, I pointed out that there were emotional Cancer Triggers that could possibly have initiated the development of cancer in your body. Let's review the personality traits that Dr. W. Douglas Brodie, M.D., observed after 30 years of work with cancer patients[226]. As your read over them, honestly ask yourself if any of these apply to you. If some of them resonate with you, that's great! Be thankful for discovering or perhaps affirming some of the emotional triggers that led you down this path.

You are moving forward and are getting a deeper understanding of what may have increased your risk factor in developing cancer. You are on the road to healing.

Circle the ones that apply to you or that you can relate to.

- Being highly conscientious, caring, dutiful, responsible, hard-working, and usually of above average intelligence.
- Exhibits a strong tendency toward carrying other people's burdens and toward taking on extra obligations, and often 'worrying for others'.
- Having a deep-seated need to make others happy. Being a 'people pleaser' with a great need for approval.
- Often lacking closeness with one or both parents, which sometimes, later in life, results in lack of closeness with spouse or others who would normally be close.
- Harbors long-suppressed toxic emotions, such as anger, resentment, and / or hostility. The cancer-susceptible individual typically internalizes such emotions and has great difficulty expressing them.
- Reacts adversely to stress and often becomes unable to cope adequately with such stress. Usually experiences an especially damaging event about 2 years before the onset of a detectable cancer.

---

226 http://www.alternative-cancer-care.com/the-cancer-personality.html

Think about the points that you circled and ask yourself how these traits may have impacted your life.

How we respond to stress is a learned habit. As children, we saw how our parents reacted to stress. Some shouted and slammed doors. Others drank to numb the pain. Some withdrew emotionally or a few may have actually had communication skills. (Consider yourself blessed if your parents had communication skills!)

More than likely, you picked up on your parents' behaviors of stress management and created some deep seated subconscious beliefs about life. In fact, between conception and the age of 5, our tiny little brains functioned at the delta and theta levels. These slower frequencies are actually 'hypnotic' and subconscious in nature. Our little brains were like sponges, and we absorbed and created our beliefs subconsciously at a very young age.

Research over the last hundred years about the emotional connection to cancer can be summed up in the 4 Ds:

- Deep anxiety.
- Deferred hope.
- Disappointment.
- Depression.

The stress behind the development of cancer may often begin at a very early age, when there are unresolved traumatic events. Those unresolved events create poor coping skills in which adult problems are not dealt with properly. This can lead to feelings of helplessness and despair.

Those very feelings impact your Immune System and your body's ability to heal.

As difficult as it may be to admit, we really do create the meaning of the various events in our lives. Thus, if we had a hand in subconsciously creating disease in our body, we invariably can also have a hand in improving our health!!

THE PLACEBO EFFECT

In order to help you understand the power of your mind and how it is involved in your healing process, let's discuss the power of the placebo.

Most of us are familiar with the 'placebo' effect, where patients are given a 'sugar pill' and told that this pill will improve their symptoms and disease. On average, about 40% -50% of people involved in a study respond favorably to a placebo.

Placebos are so powerful that they actually change the bio-chemistry of your body, which explains some of the miraculous results with placebos[227]. If you are given a placebo drug, you may believe that the researchers have your best interest at heart, which can initiate a feeling of relaxation and trust. A relaxation response is actually a biochemical and hormonal response in your body.

When you relax your mind and your body, your parasympathetic nerve system kicks in, the production of stress hormones is reduced, your Immune System works better, and happy, healing hormones are produced. This relaxed state is conducive to healing.

On the flip side, the 'nocebo' effect, demonstrates how negative beliefs affect your body. Nocebo is Latin for "I shall harm." In the book, *Love, Medicine and Miracles by Dr. Bernie Siegel*[228], Dr. Siegel describes how patients in a study for a new chemotherapy drug were given a saline solution. They were told that this 'new drug' was very powerful and could make them sick. Astonishingly, 30% of them lost their hair even though they were only receiving a saline solution.

Here's another example of the nocebo effect: In a study in France, patients were told that a particular solution would make them throw

---

227 http://www.amazon.com/Placebo-Effects-Understanding-mechanisms-disease/dp/0199559120

228 http://www.amazon.com/Love-Medicine-Miracles-Self-Healing-Exceptional-ebook/dp/B005AJQKBO/ref=sr_1_2?s=books&ie=UTF8&qid=1389287206&sr=1-2&keywords=bernie+siegel+books

up, even though it was only sugar water, and a whopping 80% of them vomited[229].

Surgeons are often wary of people who have a negative attitude about life and patients who think that they will not survive the surgery. Studies have shown that nearly 100% of patients who have a bad attitude about life and health, do die on the surgical table.

The belief that you are a victim of your genes and your DNA can have a detrimental effect on your healing. Rather than empowering themselves into believing that they can heal, many see themselves as victims, with little control on the outcome of the disease.

As was discussed in Chapter 1, your DNA is NOT your destiny. The relatively new sciences of Epigenetics and Nutrigenomics have clearly established that you can change your gene expression with specific nutrients and plant compounds.

Even more fascinating is that your DNA responds to your thoughts: positive or negative ones.

Various studies have indicated that our DNA responds to our thoughts and stress levels. Positive thoughts of love, gratitude, and joy causes the DNA strands to relax, unwind, and become longer. Stress, anger, and fear caused the DNA strands to shorten, tighten, and turn off specific protective genetic codes.

Let's examine the effect of stress on Breast Cancer.

YOUR THOUGHTS HOLD THE KEY

It is an accepted scientific fact that stress is responsible for over 80% of all diseases. The effect of emotional and psychological stress is a complex dance involving hormones, various parts of your brain, and your Immune System. Here is an oversimplification of the step by step process that leads to disease.

---

[229] Pierre Kissel and Dominique Barrucand, Placebos et Effet Placebo en Médecine (Paris: Masson, 1964)

- About 18 months to 2 years before your diagnosis, there may have been a life-changing or traumatic event that triggered intense psychological and emotional stress.
- This led to feelings of despair, hopeless, and maybe even 'giving up'.
- The emotional center of your brain, the limbic system, records and senses the emotional stress.
- The limbic system is connected to the hypothalamus and communicates the stress response through various neurochemicals and nerve pathways.
- This reaction to stress causes the hypothalamus to suppress the Immune System which allows for more growth of cancer cells.
- The hypothalamus also is connected to the pituitary gland in the brain, which is the master gland and regulator of our hormones.
- The hypothalamus communicates stress to the pituitary gland, which causes the pituitary to alter healthy hormone function. An imbalance on our hormones can create an increase in the growth and production of abnormal cells.
- Since the Immune System has been suppressed by the hypothalamus, the condition for cancer cells to multiply is set.

If this explanation has left you confused, no worries.

The important thing for you to take away from this explanation is that your Immune System and your hormones are affected by your thoughts and stress levels. Learn to think happy thoughts.

YOUR BELIEFS CREATE YOUR LIFE'S EXPERIENCE

Becoming aware of your life long beliefs and how they are affecting your health is a huge step towards healing your body. Your stress responses and certain beliefs are 'learned behaviors' that can be repaired and changed. As Laura Silva of *The Silva Method*[230] often states,:

"Your beliefs govern your living experience."

As you are on your healing journey, it is so important for you to examine your beliefs and recognize the ones that have not served you well in your life. Many times the beliefs we hold are often beliefs our parents had and we simply adopted them as truth.

What are your general beliefs about life?

- **?** Is life 'hard' and full of problems or is life an adventure and filled with joy and anticipation?
- **?** Is your home filled with stress because life is hard or is it a place of refuge and peace?
- **?** Do you believe that there is never enough money or do you see the abundance that is flowing to you?
- **?** Do you believe that most people with cancer die or do you see your body as healthy and strong?

I encourage you to get a journal and write out your thoughts about your beliefs. If you see patterns that are negative and are holding you back from enjoying your life to the fullest, then change them. It really is that easy in a sense. It's a choice!

When I was on my healing journey, I referred to my old, dysfunctional beliefs and the patterns they created as the 'Old Me'. Once I was clear about the old belief that did not serve me well, I would change the script of my old belief into a new belief. I embraced the new belief with joy and proudly affirmed that is what the 'New Me' now believes and that is how the 'New Me' feels. If I caught myself being the 'grumpy-grey Old Me', I would say, "Thank you for sharing, but the happy, sunny-bubbly, New Me believes and feels this way!"

Notice and pay attention to the energy that you attach to your beliefs. They are typically fear, shame, anger, pride, stubbornness, and

---

[230] http://mindvalley.directtrack.com/z/119/CD140/

resistance. Those energies have a very low frequency and that can keep your body stuck energetically.

E-motions are 'energy in motion'. Your emotions are a key factor in the outcome of your healing journey. Think happy thoughts of joy, gratitude, love, and peace and your body and Immune System respond in a favorable manner. Stay stuck in the dark, gloomy, negative, angry, and fearful state and your Immune System shuts down and your DNA contracts.

Your beliefs are extremely powerful. Become very clear about your beliefs, change the ones that are not supporting you, and watch your life transform before your very eyes.

There are various areas of your life that you may want to examine and heal:

- Are there any unresolved childhood events or feelings. Be honest and don't just shrug it off.
- The teenage years are full of confusion and exploration. How did you do during those years?
- As a young adult, did you make good choices? Did you begin to create patterns that were dysfunctional but had no idea how to change them?
- Did you raise a family and pass on those 'beliefs' about life to your children? Did you teach them joy and laughter and gratitude or were you an example of bitterness, anger, and frustration? If you feel guilty about any parental mistakes, don't beat yourself up about it because we ALL have goofed up somehow. You did the best you knew how with the information you had. If there are unresolved issues with your children, deal with them now with love, humility, and kindness. Ask for forgiveness and tell them you are sorry. Remind them how much you love them.
- How is your relationship with your significant other?
- Do you have a circle of friends that support and nurture you or are they negative and not trustworthy? Are you able to draw boundaries, especially during this time of healing?

If you are serious about changing your beliefs and healing your emotional wounds, there are 2 programs that I highly recommend.

- *Silva Mind Body Healing*[231]: This is a CD program that examines every aspect of health and teaches you that YOU have control of your mind and body. You can learn to train your mind to serve you better and to heal very deep, old wounds. This program guides you through the various factors that have hindered your health and teaches you how to visualize and FEEL your body as healthy, whole, and complete. The meditations include alpha and theta frequency sounds to help calm your body and mind.
- *Getting Well Again*[232] by Dr. Carl Simonton is a book written by a radiation oncologist. As he worked with cancer patients he recognized that those who had a positive attitude and a 'will to live' because of a goal or an event that they were looking forward to, would generally recover or have fewer side effects to the treatments. He began to teach his patients how to visualize their Immune System attacking the cancer and invited them to look at the emotional 'payback' of the cancer. His statistics of overall survival rates with his patients indicate the power of the mind-body connection in healing the body.

DID YOU TAKE YOUR HAPPY PILL TODAY?

I am not talking about an anti-depressant. I am talking about making a conscious effort to be happy and to plan activities that create more endorphins. Most people have not learned that *Happy is Normal*. What is NOT normal is that too many of us live our lives, day after day, living life very unconsciously. We take so many things for granted and focus on the negative events. We let our mind wander to all the 'what ifs' and the 'should haves' rather than focusing on the outcomes that we want.

---

[231] http://mindvalley.directtrack.com/z/119/CD140/

[232] http://amzn.com/0553280333

It's not rocket science that happy people are generally healthier and live longer than those that are depressed and gloomy. ***It has been stated that happiness can be compared to the psychological equivalent of Vitamin C[233].*** Happy people have fewer stress hormones and a stronger Immune System. Affirming your personal, happy beliefs buffers and protects you against the stress response that weakens your Immune System[234]. (Remember how psychological stress affects your hormones and Immune System?)

How do we define happiness as human beings on this planet? According to Dictionary.com[235], happiness is characterized by or an indication of, pleasure, contentment, or joy. Can practicing happiness actually increase your life span?

An interesting study called 'The Nun Study' examined old diaries of Catholic nuns that were born before 1917[236]. In their early twenties, they were asked to keep a journal and an autobiography of their lives. Fifty years later, researchers examined the journals to find that the nuns that wrote about joy and a fulfilled life lived nearly 10 years longer that the nuns who complained and expressed negative thoughts.

At first, it may feel challenging to feel happy about this cancer that is growing in your body but as you understand more about your beliefs and how they may have contributed to your stress levels and impairment of your Immune System, the easier it will get.

It becomes very empowering to know that you do have quite a measure of control over your health and body!

If you have struggled with happiness and joy, here are a few things that may help your let go of that grumpy-grey Grinch inside of you.

- What is YOUR great purpose?
- Develop a spiritual connection with God (Jehovah), your Creator or Universal Energy, whatever it is for you. I believe

---

233 http://science.howstuffworks.com/life/happy-people-live-longer.htm
234 http://www.ncbi.nlm.nih.gov/pubmed/16262767
235 http://dictionary.reference.com/browse/happy
236 http://www.ncbi.nlm.nih.gov/pubmed/11374751

that we all have a purpose and if we live our lives fully and completely, we honor our Creator with our lives. If you consider yourself a spiritual person and feel connected to God, spend time in prayer, asking for strength and direction. If you don't feel very connected and are not sure about your spiritual beliefs, spend time exploring that, reading various books on spirituality. Finding YOUR greater purpose in this life can be very assuring and calming.

- Meditate every day.
- Monks who spend years meditating have a larger left prefrontal cortex, the part of the brain that is responsible for happiness. You don't have to spend hours meditating. Simply 20 minutes per day has proven to create very positive results in the brain. Research shows that regular meditation can actually permanently 're-wire' your brain for improved levels of happiness. With a little time and effort, happiness can become a learned behavior and a regular part of your life.

I've always been attracted to meditation because I experienced the benefits of it at a very young age. At the age of 18, I was introduced to Transcendental Meditation and certainly benefited from the relaxation that it gave me at that time in my life. As an avid runner for over 40 years, running and jogging is a form of meditation for me. When I was on my healing journey, I found it extremely beneficial to block out time every day to meditate.

Visualizing a positive outcome of your journey and 'seeing' and 'feeling' your body as healthy, whole, and complete is extremely powerful.

Meditation creates mental, emotional, and physical benefits. A study conducted at the Massachusetts General Hospital by a Dr. Gaelle Desbordes found that people who meditated as little as 20 minutes per day showed changes in the area of the brain which regulates emotions. Basically, these changes improved happiness and decreased depression. Be open to making time in your life for this mental and emotional 'exercise'.

Create a quiet spot in your home. Light a candle. Rub some essential oils on your neck and forehead. Breathe slowly and relax.

LOOK FORWARD TO SOMETHING

Think about your future and create a visual image about something that would give you pleasure. It can be as simple as going to the movies or taking a vacation to the beach or mountains. How about a night out with the girls? A massage or spa day? Like to garden or paint? All these activities raise your endorphin levels and the human growth hormone that keeps the body young and healthy.

Simply the anticipation of watching a funny movie has been shown to raise endorphin production by 27% and the human growth hormone by 87%[237]!

CREATE A POSITIVE ENVIRONMENT IN YOUR HOME

We spend a lot of time in our homes. Create an environment that reflects life, calm, and nature. A few green plants, occasional fresh flowers, candles, and soft music stimulates the parasympathetic nerve system and the relaxation hormones that are conducive to healing.

MAKE SOMEONE SMILE TODAY

People who commit acts of kindness tend to be happier and have lower levels of stress hormones in their body. You might be thinking, "Well, I am the one in need of an act of kindness, since I am the one dealing with cancer." No matter how dire or dark your situation may feel, calling a friend in need, sending a thank you note, giving a much needed hug will only lighten and improve your mood. There truly is more joy in giving than in receiving.

---

[237] http://phys.org/news63293074.html

MOVE YOUR BODY

Moving your body produces a type of neurotransmitter called endorphins. They are produced by the pituitary gland and the hypothalamus during exercise and sexual activity. Endorphins produce a euphoric feeling and can also block the transmission of pain[238]. Choose what makes you feel good: walk, bounce on your rebounder, ride a bike, hike, yoga, tai-chi, etc. The important thing is that you move your body.

If you are physically not able to move your body or feel too weak to exercise, then meditate and visual yourself doing your favorite activity. Put some emotion behind it and really *feel* yourself doing the exercise. You will gain benefits just from thinking about your body moving.

If you are lying in bed, move your arms and legs for a few minutes. Any activity is beneficial!

LEARN HOW TO BREATHE

On average, we breathe anywhere from 17,000 to 28,000 breaths per day. The majority of the time, we do so unconsciously without paying much attention to it. The very action of breathing involves taking in oxygen and expelling carbon dioxide and other gaseous toxins.

The more often you take the time to medicate, the more you will become conscious of deep breathing. Most of us are shallow breathers, especially when we are feeling stressed. Learning to fill your lungs with air has many benefits.

First of all, deep breathing is very calming and centering. It gets you to slow down and become aware of the moment you are in. It is very cleansing. In her book, *Molecules of Emotions*[239], Dr. Candace Pert states that: "The peptide-respiratory link is well documented. (Peptides are amino acid chains that purify, create

---

238 http://science.howstuffworks.com/life/exercise-happiness2.htm
239 http://candacepert.com/

antibodies, and signal hormonal changes.) Virtually any peptide found anywhere else can be found in the respiratory system. This peptide substrate may provide the scientific rationale for the *powerful healing effects of consciously controlled breathing patterns.*"

BE GRATEFUL

It might seem difficult to feel grateful about this healing journey and all that you have been through so far. As I mentioned earlier, you have a choice to be bitter or to be better.

As I experienced my healing journey, learning to be better was a huge part of my healing. I was determined that I would truly get to the core of my health challenges once and for all. I chose to see my experience as a gift and not a burden.

As Dr. Simonton so beautifully expresses, cancer is a message of love. Your body has been whispering to you for years but did not get your attention. Now it is screaming at you and telling you to change and to take responsibility for your health. It is telling you to love your body. To be kind to your body; to rest, nurture, nourish, detox, and heal.

Be grateful for all the new insights you have gained since you were diagnosed. Be grateful for your doctors and the technology that discovered the cancer.

Be grateful for the organic foods that are available to you.

Be grateful for the knowledge that your cancer coach is sharing with you.

Be grateful for your body's ability to heal.

Be grateful for fresh air and a blue sky. Be grateful for the rain.

Be grateful for the positive relationships in your life.

I think you get the point.

Learn to live your life consciously. Keep a journal by your bed and write down everything for which you are grateful. This increases your awareness about gratitude. It helps you appreciate the bountiful life you have in so many ways. The very act of writing these thoughts is very therapeutic and calming.

There are many avenues to help you heal your emotional wounds. There is the typical psychotherapy and counseling with a psychologist and therapist. There is also an emerging therapy called 'Energy Psychology' that connects the mind with the body during the therapy sessions.

Examples of these therapies are German New Medicine, Emotional Freedom Technique (EFT), Rapid Eye Technology, Heart Math, The Emotion Code, and many others.

Do your research and pick something that resonates with you. Many of these therapies can be conducted in the comfort of your home.

To see an example of an EFT video about releasing the emotions involved with Breast Cancer, visit this link on my web site[240].

I believe Dr. Candace Pert[241] said it best,

"Most psychologists treat the mind as disembodied, a phenomenon with little or no connection to the physical body. Conversely, physicians treat the body with no regard to the mind or the emotions. But the body and the mind are not separate and we cannot treat one without the other."

I will close this chapter on emotional healing with some thoughts from a palliative nurse who worked with dying people for many years. What she has to say is quite sobering and comforting at the same time. ***She found that there were 5 main regrets that people had about their life[242].*** Don't' let this be you. Live your life to the fullest every day so when that day comes when you do take your last breath and go to sleep, you will do so feeling grateful that you served your purpose and that your mission was accomplished.

---

240 http://breastcancerconqueror.com/videos/

241 http://candacepert.com/

242 http://www.ariseindiaforum.org/nurse-reveals-the-top-5-regrets-people-make-on-their-deathbed/

- I wish I'd had the courage to live a life true to myself, not the life others expected of me.
- I wish I didn't work so hard.
- I wish I'd had the courage to express my feelings.
- I wish I had stayed in touch with my friends.
- I wish I had let myself be happier.
-

POINTS TO PONDER

- Healing my emotional wounds is an important part of my physical healing.
- What kind of attitude will I have about this cancer?
- The message of cancer can be a message of love.
- Change is part of the healing process.
- Do I have a 'cancer personality'?
- How I react to stress and events in my life is a learned habit. If it was learned, it can be 'unlearned'.
- My mind is a very powerful tool in my healing.
- My mind can create bio-chemical reactions for my good or for my detriment. I get to choose.
- My DNA is NOT my destiny. I can change my gene expression and turn on healthy genes through improved nutrition and specific supplements.
- My positive thoughts create a cascading effect of healthy hormones and an improved Immune System.
- My beliefs create my living experience.
- I can learn how to be happy and to improve my happiness level.
- Meditation and exercise have many beneficial effects on my mind, body, and Immune System
- Deep breathing is cleansing, comforting, and grounding.

- Energy Psychology tools are very effective in dealing with the mind-body connection for improved health.
- I choose to live my life with no regrets.

YOUR HEALING JOURNEY ACTION STEPS

- Examine the Cancer Personality profile and determine what areas call for improvement in my life.
- Express your thoughts in your journal about what you believe may be your emotional connection to the Breast Cancer.
- Order the book *Getting Well Again* by Dr. Carl Simonton. Commit to reading it and doing the exercises he recommends.
- Order a meditation program that deals with the mind body connection and meditate every day for no less than 15 minutes. Make the time to meditate more frequently throughout the day.
- Happiness is a choice. I chose to be happy today. Happy is my new normal.
- Happiness can become a learned habit. I can incorporate daily habits to improve my happiness levels.
- Become conscious of deep breathing several times throughout the day.
- I choose to live my life without regret.

CHAPTER 6

ESSENTIAL #5 EMBRACE BIOLOGICAL DENTISTRY

"Healing takes courage and we all have courage, even if we have to dig a little to find it."

~

Tori Amos

I discovered the dental connection to health and disease very early in my career in the early 80s. I was fascinated to learn that the so-called 'silver' fillings were a hodgepodge of toxic metals that were slowly releasing toxins into the body, taxing the Immune System, and affecting the neurological system. In my 35 years of experience in the Wellness Industry, I would have to say that I witnessed 9 out of 10 patients having adverse effects to their health as a result of dental toxicities.

If you truly want to heal your body, you **must** address the dental issues. Can you recover from Breast Cancer without addressing the issue? Maybe. But I will say that your chances of overcoming cancer are much greater if you address the dental toxicities.

If you absolutely cannot confront this issue head on, then the next best step is to implement homeopathic remedies and specific nutrients that help to detoxify heavy metals from the body. More on this later.

Obviously I am not a dentist and am not representing myself as one. However, the information that is presented here is a growing movement called Biological Dentistry. In my opinion, the pioneers in this field were Dr. Weston Price and Dr. Hal Huggins.

In the early 1900s, Dr. Price was way ahead of his time by theorizing that there was a relationship between dental health and physical health. He discovered extremely toxic bacteria in root canals and infected gums and concluded that these bacteria created a serious toxic load in the body. By injecting bacteria from a root canal into laboratory animals, he was able to replicate the same diseases the human donor had in about 80% to 100% of the animals.

In the 1980s, Dr. Hal Huggins, a Colorado dentist, began promoting a safer, alternative method to traditional dentistry called 'biological dentistry'. ***The principle behind biological dentistry was the safe removal of toxic metals and root canals which were then replaced with compatible, non-reactive compounds.*** Before having any metals replaced, he encouraged his patients to have a 'serum compatibility' blood test done, in order to determine what dental compounds were safe to use for that particular patient. You can compare it to an 'allergy' test for your teeth and Immune System.

This is a procedure that I had done back in the early 90s, and I encourage you to begin your dental 'clean up' with this blood test as well. If you only have 1-2 fillings that need replacing, it is not as serious of an issue. But I would encourage you to consider this test if you have over 3 amalgams that need replacing. There are 2 labs in Colorado that specialize in dental material reactivity testing Clifford Consulting and Research[243] and Biocomp Laboratories, Inc.[244]

---

[243] http://www.ccrlab.com/

[244] http://www.biocomplabs.com/index.html

THAT'S NOT SILVER IN YOUR MOUTH

According to the research provided by Dr.Tom McGuire[245], a mercury free dentist who has a plethora of information about safe dentistry, amalgams consist of 50% elemental mercury. On a global scale, over 400 tons of mercury is placed in people's mouths each year!

At room temperature, mercury vapors are released from amalgams, so imagine what happens when the amalgam sits in your mouth at 98° degrees Fahrenheit or when you are enjoying that hot cup of tea!

Mercury vapors are also released with a small amount of friction such as chewing and brushing your teeth.

You have to understand one thing about mercury: there is NO safe level of mercury.

One single atom of mercury has proven to be toxic. Based on very conservative estimates, over 67 million Americans exceed the 'safe' level of exposure established by the EPA.

How does mercury impact your health? Here is an oversimplification of the symptoms created by amalgams because essentially, mercury impacts every system in your body:

- It impacts your digestive system and causes everything from colitis to constipation.
- Since mercury is classified as a neurotoxin, it can affect your mental and emotional health. Mercury has been linked to depression, anxiety, and even hallucinations. It also causes learning disorders, tremors, numbness, and memory loss.
- By poisoning your endocrine system, mercury toxicity can lead to Chronic Fatigue.

---

[245] http://dentalwellness4u.com/index.html

- Chronic exposure to a deadly toxin will trigger chronic inflammation in the body, which is a precursor to so many diseases, especially cancer.
- Amalgams may make you more sensitive to EMFs. As we discussed in Chapter 3: Reduce Your Toxic Exposure, EMFs pose a serious threat to our environment and our health. The metals in your mouth can act as 'antenna' that attract EMFs to your body and especially to your brain. If you have gold fillings and amalgams in your mouth, a galvanic electro-current is created, causing serious erosion to the amalgam and thus releasing much more vapor into your body[246].

THE DENTAL – BREAST CANCER CONNECTION

According to the Journal of Applied Toxicology, metallo-estrogens are an emerging class of estrogens with potential to add to the estrogen burden of breast tissue, ultimately leading to an increased risk of Breast Cancer[247].

The critical issue here is that mercury and other heavy metals used in dentistry can be classified as metallo-estrogens: metals that bind to estrogen receptors and mimic estrogen. These metals are a new class of cancer-causing estrogens. Research has confirmed that excess dietary cadmium, for example, mimics estrogen and can lead to the development of estrogen-dependent malignancies[248]. (Cadmium is often found in trace amounts in amalgams and dental materials.)

Mercury significantly stimulates the growth of MCF-7 Breast Cancer cells, which are found in Invasive Breast Ductal Carcinoma and are typically estrogen and progesterone positive[249].

In 2011, a Canadian research team assessed Breast Cancer tissue biopsies and found a significant accumulation of heavy metals, such as mercury, zinc, and nickel in the diseased tissue[250].

---

246 http://orthomolecular.org/library/jom/1983/pdf/1983-v12n03-p184.pdf
247 http://www.ncbi.nlm.nih.gov/pubmed/16489580
248 http://www.ncbi.nlm.nih.gov/pubmed/22422990
249 http://www.ncbi.nlm.nih.gov/pubmed/15712295

ROOT CANALS – INFECTED TOXIC LOADS

Think about this: if you had a dead and infected gall bladder or appendix in your body, how sick would that make you? Very! In fact, you could die from the systemic infection that it would cause.

Root canals are no different. Your teeth are living entities that can become very diseased and infected. ***No matter how aseptic a dentist may try to make that tooth, it is a dead tissue that creates a toxic focal site.*** I can't tell you how many thermograms I have seen with a hot red spot in the area of a root canal, which is often on the same side as the Breast Cancer.

When a dentist performs root canal therapy, his goal is to remove the nerve tissue, blood vessels, and other tissue from the pulp chamber and root canal. He will use a small file and a series of irrigating solutions like sodium hypochlorite (bleach), to try to decontaminate the tissue. Once the canal is visually clean, he will insert fillings such as cements or epoxy resins which may contain Bisphenol A, an estrogenic compound that has been shown to stimulate normal breast cells to behave like cancer cells[251].

But if you go back to Dental Anatomy 101, the roots of your teeth are implanted into the jaw bone and are held in place by tiny ligaments. There are literally miles of tiny tubules and blood vessels attached to each root. Filing and irrigating the large root chamber does not touch any of these tiny tubules which are a haven for all types of bacteria.

No matter how aseptic a dentist may try to make that tooth, there is always a pocket of anaerobic toxic bacteria that forms at the base of the root.

These bacteria drip potent and pathogenic toxins into your circulatory and lymphatic system. This dead tooth may sit in your jaw for years, without any obvious symptoms like tooth pain, but in the

---

[250] http://www.ncbi.nlm.nih.gov/pubmed/16804515
[251] http://breastcancerconqueror.com/bpa-and-breast-cancer/

meantime it is weakening your Immune System and contributing to inflammatory and auto-immune diseases.

In a 5 year study, Dr. Robert Jones, a researcher of the relationship between root canals and Breast Cancer, found that 93% of women with Breast Cancer had 1 or more root canals[252].

Dr. Josef Issels, M.D., a German M.D. who treated thousands of cancer patients for 40 years, found that 97% of his cancer patients had root canal-filled teeth[253].

The Paracelsus Cancer Clinic in Switzerland found that 98% of Breast Cancer patients had 1 or more root canals on the same meridian as the original breast tumor[254].

The Toxic Element Research Foundation (TERF[255]), a non-profit research foundation, used state of the art DNA testing and identified 42 different species of anaerobic bacteria in root canal samples. These bacterial toxins are associated with many auto-immune diseases, cardiovascular disease, and neurological issues.

It is an established medical fact that chronic infections can contribute to the development of cancer by creating inflammatory responses and biochemical changes in the body. In fact, several bacterial toxins interfere with healthy cell communication in a way that promotes tumor growth[256].

From this information, the chemical and biological impact of amalgams, root canals, and dental implants on your health is quite clear. However, there is also the energetic aspect to consider.

Your Acupuncture Meridian System is a distribution network of your CHI or life force. This system is independent of the nerves, blood, and lymphatic systems and yet ties all of your organs and systems together. This principle is very important for you to understand since

---

252 http://breastcancerconqueror.com/is-your-root-canal-increasing-your-risk-for-breast-cancer/

253 http://www.issels.com/history.aspx#sthash.If6QomJa.dpbs

254 http://www.new-cancer-treatments.org/Articles/RootCanals.html

255 http://terfinfo.com/

256 http://www.ncbi.nlm.nih.gov/pubmed/12088666

the meridians that affect the breast are also connected to specific teeth, namely the 4th and 5th teeth from your center tooth, right and left, top and bottom. Additionally, on the upper jaw, the molars, or the 6th and 7th teeth from the center tooth, are also associated with the breast meridian.

Take a look at the excellent dental-meridian chart complied by Dr. Ralph Wilson of NeuralTherapy.com[257].

This life energy in the meridian system travels in cycles every 24 hours and flows through ALL your organs and teeth. However, if there is a hunk of metal, root canal, or implant in a tooth, that CHI energy can be 'short-circuited' and reduced. Over a period of time, this may have an adverse effect on the organ that is attached to that tooth.

When I was in active practice and tested my patients with Bio-Energetic Screenings, I repeatedly found dental issues connected to serious health problems, including cancer.

CAVITATIONS

A cavitation is an infection of the bone caused by periodontal ligaments not being properly extracted after a tooth is pulled. When the membranes are left behind, an infected focal site is created, even if the hole closes over and is sealed. With time, this causes sponginess in the bone and bone erosion.

But the more serious issue is that this cavitation is a breeding ground for toxic bacteria. This is a very similar scenario as the root canal issue. Not only does the cavitation release deadly toxins into the lymphatic and circulatory system, but it can also affect the meridian flow at that particular meridian.

If you have ever had an extraction, consider having that site examined by an experienced Biological Dentist.

---

257 http://www.isisboston.com/assets/PDF-Files/Tooth-Organ-Chart.pdf

DENTAL IMPLANTS

I would NEVER have a dental implant screwed into my jaw bone. Think about the implications of that procedure. First of all, the metals used in implants can be a hodgepodge of metals such as titanium, nickel, chromium, aluminum, vanadium, etc. Many people have allergic reactions to metals implanted into their body. Secondly, the implant is drilled into your jaw bone, often causing severe infections, nerve damage, and chronic pain.

Auto-immune issues can be sparked or aggravated with this foreign metal permanently implanted into the jaw. Just as amalgams cause a galvanic, electrical response in the body, implants can to the same. Lastly, the metal implant will most definitely interfere with the flow of energy in your meridian system.

As you can see, your dental health has a huge impact on your overall health. Only consult with the best when it comes to your health. That is why I always refer my clients to Biological Dentists.

BIOLOGICAL DENTISTS TO THE RESCUE

What makes a Biological Dentist (BD) different from a regular dentist? A BD appreciates that materials in your teeth and diseases in your mouth have long lasting effects on your health. BDs understand the concepts of natural healing and often work with other like-minded health care providers for the benefit of the patient. Through various forms of testing, whether it is blood serum, allergy testing, or Bio-energetic testing, a BD will determine what materials are most compatible and safe for a patient.

Unfortunately, I have witnessed too many cases of dentists that 'claim' they are BDs, but don't align themselves with the true philosophy and care of Biological Dentistry. Often, they have not had the proper training and do not use the proper equipment and protocols.

Here is a list of questions to ask a BD before you sit in the dental chair and open your mouth:

- Are you truly a mercury-free practice? If so, for how long?
- Where did you get your training?

- Do you belong to any professional Biological Dentist organizations? If so, which one?
- Before you consider removing amalgams, do you use an amalgameter to read the electrical charge on the tooth to see which quadrant needs primary attention?
- Do you recommend serum compatibility testing to determine what materials can be used that will not cause an allergic reaction? If not, do you test material with bio-energetic equipment?
- Do you have specialized equipment such as high speed suction and mercury vapor collectors and filters?
- Do you provide a nose piece for Oxygen while the amalgam is being removed?
- Do you use a rubber dam to prevent any spillage of mercury on the tongue or in the mouth?
- Do you recommend a heavy metal detoxification program after the removal of the amalgams?
- Are you familiar with cavitations? If so, how do you treat them?

Here is a list of organizations and non-profit groups that support Biological Dentistry.

International Academy of Biological Dentistry and Medicine

www.iabdm.org

Holistic Dental Association

www.holisticdental.org

Dental Amalgam Mercury Solutions

www.amalgam.org

Dental Wellness Institute

www.dentalwellness4u.com

DENTAL DETOX

As soon as you understand the dental connection to health and disease, it's time to start detoxing the heavy metals that have accumulated in your body. As discussed in Chapter 3 - Reduce Your Toxic Exposure, there are many ways to detox. Here are a few simple ways to specifically address the dental detox:

- Chlorella is a fresh water algae that has been shown to eliminate methyl mercury in the bodies of laboratory animals.[258] It is best to find a chlorella that has a 'broken cell wall' which improves its digestibility. A very reliable and clean source is Sun Chlorella[259]. Start slowly and increase to the point where you are using 4 grams (about 1 teaspoon) of chlorella each day.
- Increase your glutathione levels with raw whey protein[260] or with a product called Enduracell, which is a broccoli sprout powder[261] high in Sulforaphane.
- Cilantro tincture can be taken orally or applied to the wrists twice per day.
- Use specific homeopathic formulas designed to stimulate the body to expel heavy metals.

POINTS TO PONDER

- If you truly want to heal your body, the dental connection has to be addressed.
- Infected teeth and gums can create disease in other organs.
- Amalgams are 50% mercury.
- Mercury is the most toxic metal on the planet.

---

[258] https://www.jstage.jst.go.jp/result?cdjournal=jts&item1=4&word1=methyl+mercury+and+chlorella

[259] http://breastcancerconquerorshop.com/product/chlorella/

[260] http://breastcancerconquerorshop.com/product/one-world-whey-vanilla-1-lb/

[261] http://breastcancerconquerorshop.com/product/broccoli-sprout-powder/

- Heating amalgams to body temperature release toxic mercury vapors.
- Brushing amalgams with a tooth brush releases toxic mercury vapors.
- Mercury and other metals stimulate the growth of Breast Cancer cells by acting as metallo-estrogens.
- A root canal-filled tooth drips bacterial toxins into the body.
- 93% or more women with Breast Cancer also have root canals.
- Metals in your teeth and jaw may weaken your life force or CHI that travels through your meridian system, directly affecting specific organs.
- Biological Dentists understand the dental connection to health and are trained to remove any toxic materials in your mouth.

YOUR HEALING JOURNEY ACTION STEPS

- ➢ Take inventory of how many amalgams and root canals you have.
- ➢ Examine the Meridian – Dental Chart provided by NeuralTherapy.com[262] and determine what organs may be affected with your present dental situation.
- ➢ Find a biological dentist (BD) in your area by using the suggested websites.
- ➢ Make sure to interview the dentist using the 10 questions in this chapter before you allow them to work in your mouth. It is YOUR health and YOUR body.
- ➢ Begin a dental detox if you presently have metals in your mouth or if you ever had metals in your mouth.

---

262 http://www.isisboston.com/assets/PDF-Files/Tooth-Organ-Chart.pdf

CHAPTER 7

ESSENTIAL #6
REPAIR YOUR BODY WITH THERAPEUTIC PLANTS

"The art of healing comes from nature, not from the physician. Therefore the physician must start from nature."

~

Paracelsus

This step is what seems to cause the most confusion and frustration with women. There is a maze of information on the Internet about the latest and greatest 'cancer cures' that claim that their products work best.

When I began my healing journey, I had seen firsthand how patients responded to various protocols, so I had a pretty good idea about which direction I would go. But even with decades of experience and research under my belt, I still found it daunting to sift through all the various products and pick a protocol that would work best for me.

Fortunately, I was able to test my products Bio-energetically to make sure that they were compatible and were, in fact, going to be effective for me.

In this chapter, I will only discuss the products and protocols that *I have had personal experience with.* There are literally hundreds of various products and protocols that have proven successful but not all remedies and programs work for everyone.

There is no 'one-size-fits-all' protocol that guarantees success 100% of the time.

You might have the best products and herbs but if your emotions or hormones are out of balance, the products may not be as effective. Each and every essential has to be applied successfully in order for the body to have the capacity to truly heal.

In my personal healing journey, I used a combination of 4 main categories:

- **Tumor Terminators** to weaken the cancer cells
- **Body Builders** that boost your Immune System
- **Nourishing Nutrients** that support your healing process
- **Favorite Foods** that weaken cancer

It would be impossible to list all of the combinations of nutrients and herbs that have proven successful in healing the body. Do your research and work with a qualified and licensed practitioner that has experience in successfully working with cancer patients. If you can, have your products tested Bio-energetically with an EAV machine to make sure that your products are compatible with your body.

TUMOR TERMINATORS

Nature has gifted us with innumerable supportive plants and herbs to help heal the body and boost the Immune System. Many of these have been scientifically proven to target and kill cancer cells, while not harming healthy cells. I like to refer to some of the phytochemicals as 'herbal chemotherapy'. The beauty of this 'herbal chemo' is that it is efficient, non-toxic, and causes apoptosis (death of the cell) to cancer cells only.

I don't want you to simply take my word about the power of natural medicine. I want you to take the time to go to ***www.usa.gov*** or the National Library of Medicine and search for 'Herbal Breast Cancer Apoptosis'.

You will see over 32,000 published studies about natural medicines that kill Breast Cancer cells!

Let's take a look at what makes cancer cells unique and what it takes to weaken and destroy them.

When healthy, normal cells begin to age or develop DNA damage, they secrete a protein that causes them to self-destruct[263]. They are then replaced with younger, healthier cells.

Cancer cells, on the other hand, have mutated, which disrupts the self-destruction pathway. They produce a protein called 'survivin' that prevents them from dying, thus they no longer have that built in mechanism that causes them to self-destruct[264]. Despite growth inhibiting signals that are sent from adjacent cells to stop reproducing, cancer cells turn a deaf ear and keep growing.

Some types of cancers even begin to create their own blood flow (angiogenesis) so they can have an ample supply of food and nourishment. ***Trying to kill cancer cells by creating DNA damage with toxic chemicals and radiation is very counter-productive since cancer cells resist dying in many ways.***

But what creates a cancer cell to begin with? Typically it begins with some sort of mutation or DNA damage as a result of foreign chemicals, radiation, or free radicals. A healthy cell would self-repair or self-destruct at this point, but a cancer cells slips through the repair process and also escapes our Immune System's watchful eye. If it keeps ignoring the growth inhibiting signals, it starts to duplicate and replicate.

---

263 http://www.disabled-world.com/health/cancer/treatment/cancer-cells.php
264 http://en.wikipedia.org/wiki/Survivin

There are various aspects of your Immune System that track down, devour, and destroy cancer cells. However, cancer cells have the ability to 'trick' the Immune System by maintaining specific proteins found on the surface of a healthy cell, thereby escaping the attack of the Immune System. Cancer cells also produce certain enzymes that sabotage the Immune System by putting it to sleep.

Chemotherapy and radiation treatments attempt to kill the cancer cells but, unfortunately, cancer cells are very resistive. Too many times the patients do not die from the cancer, but they die as a result of the toxic therapies.

According to the National Institute of Health, 65% of cancer patients who responded to a 2007 survey had used complementary approaches for immune enhancement, pain management, and general wellness[265]. The NIH recognizes that there is a paradigm shift that is occurring and people want more control over how they manage their health issues.

Mainstream medicine and Big Pharma turn the other cheek when it comes to promoting and encouraging the use of natural medicines. There is no money to be made in promoting herbal products since you can't patent a plant. Unfortunately the cancer industry is more interested in profits than standing up for the REAL cause and cure for cancer. Hundreds of thousands, if not millions of people have turned their health around with lifestyle changes by incorporating the power of natural medicines in their life.

Here is an alphabetical list and description of some of the natural medicines that can act as **Tumor Terminators.**

BLOOD ROOT AND PROTEOLYTIC ENZYMES

Blood root is a perennial plant native to North America that has 'blood red' roots; thus, the name Blood Root. The power of this herb is a special plant alkaloid called Sanguinarine[266]. Sanguinarine weakens the 'survivin' protein that keeps cancer cells from dying; therefore, it

---

[265] http://nccam.nih.gov/health/cancer/camcancer.htm
[266] http://www.ncbi.nlm.nih.gov/pmc/articles/PMC2996866/

induces apoptosis or cancer cell suicide. The beauty of this is that it does not kill healthy cells but only targets cancer cells. I find this mechanism miraculous!

Sanguinarine is anti-inflammatory and has many anti-cancer properties. One important property is that it inhibits the Vascular Epithelial Growth Factor (VEGF) in Breast Cancer cells[267]. This is a very important factor since many solid tumors create their own blood flow to keep 'feeding' the tumor. If you can stop the VEGF from being produced, the tumor has less of a chance of surviving.

One of the leading causes of death with Breast Cancer is the spread of cancer cells or metastasis.

Sanguinarine has powerful anti-metastatic properties that inhibit and suppress Breast Cancer cells' migration and invasion[268].

High doses of pancreatic enzymes are an essential part of the blood root protocol or any cancer protocol. The thought of healing cancer with enzyme therapy was first discovered by Dr. John Beard, an embryologist involved in cancer research back in the early 1900s. He discovered that cancer patients' blood samples were extremely deficient in pancreatic enzymes. His Trophoblast Theory of Cancer is very interesting[269]:

Being an embryologist, Beard had a light bulb moment when he realized that the fetal placenta was very similar to cancer cells. Placental cells:

- Are very primitive.
- They divide and multiply uncontrollably.
- They create their own blood flow.
- They invade the healthy tissue of the uterine wall.

---

267 http://www.ncbi.nlm.nih.gov/pmc/articles/PMC3673330/
268 http://www.ncbi.nlm.nih.gov/pubmed/24220687
269 http://www.greenmedinfo.com/affiliate/2929/node/109251

Theoretically, if there was not a specific trigger mechanism to stop the placenta from growing, it would continue to spread and invade other tissues. So what was the trigger that stopped the growth of the placenta?

Pancreatic Enzymes produced by the fetus!

The day that the fetus began to produce and secrete pancreatic enzymes, day 56, the placenta stopped growing.

So what are enzymes? Enzymes are biological catalysts that accelerate reactions and permit certain reactions from occurring. Some enzymes attack proteins while some others attack carbohydrates. Enzymes attach themselves to white blood cells, using them as a means of transportation. Since the outer membrane of the cancer cell is very tough and fibrous, it makes it very difficult for anything to penetrate the cell. (Another reason why chemotherapy is not very effective)

Pancreatic enzymes have the ability to destroy the carbohydrate chain and protein layers in the fibrin of the cancer cell wall, thus, making the cancer cell more vulnerable and weaker.

Scientists who researched the effectiveness of enzyme therapy in a 2005 study came to very promising conclusions[270]:

- The mixture of these enzymatic activities produces potent anti-metastatic and anti-tumor effects in cellular, animal, and human systems.
- The treatment of cultured tumor cells with enzymes causes complete arrest of the directional movement of metastatic cells.
- These findings support the conclusion that proteolysis (the breakdown of the cancer cell wall) is the active mechanism of the proenzyme treatment.
- Proenzyme therapy shows remarkable selective effects that result in growth inhibition of tumor cells with metastatic potential.

---

[270] http://cancerx.org/Enzyme%20NOVAK-TRNKA.pdf

The key to success in enzyme therapy is reaching saturation. Saturation is reached by taking enzymes in frequent and large doses. Saturation with enzyme therapy is described as a distinct burning, itching sensation around the anus. Since there are dead skin cells near the anus, enzymes will 'digest' the proteins from these dead or defective cells. Once you feel that sensation, it is an indication that your blood stream is saturated with the enzymes, which is a great thing.

Another key enzyme in healing your body is Bromelain. Bromelain is an enzyme found in pineapple stems and immature fruits of pineapples. Bromelain was found to be more effective in killing cancer cells than a chemotherapy agent[271]. In a 2012 study, Bromelain was reported to promote apoptosis, (cancer cell death), in Breast Cancer cells[272].

B 17 AND APRICOT SEEDS

In the early 70s, a 5 year trial was quietly underway in the most prestigious cancer research center in the United States: Memorial Sloan-Kettering Cancer Center in New York City. It was headed by a Dr. Kanematsu Sugiura[273], a well-respected cancer researcher. The research subject was Laetrile, which is the chemically modified form of B 17 or amygdalin, and its effect on cancer.

Dr. Sugiura came to 5 conclusions on the effect of Laetrile on laboratory mice[274]:

- It improved the general health of the mice.
- It appeared to relieve their pain.
- It inhibited the growth of tumors.
- It stopped the spread of tumors.
- It acted as a cancer prevention.

---

271 http://www.ncbi.nlm.nih.gov/pubmed/17893836
272 http://www.ncbi.nlm.nih.gov/pubmed/22191568
273 http://www.whale.to/cancer/sugiura_h.html
274 http://www.whale.to/cancer/sugiura_h.html

Dr. Sugiura found that when he used laetrile on cancerous mice, 77% of them did not develop a spread of the disease. He took his findings to his superiors, but his reports and studies were never published. Hmmmm....

If this supplement was found to be so effective against cancer, why is it not readily available for use?

The story of apricot kernels takes us to a remote kingdom in the Himalayan Mountains called Hunza. Hunzacuts are well known to live beyond 100 plus years, cancer-free, and living their life in good health. Interestingly, their diet contains over 200 times the amount of nitrilosides, (which contains B 17), compared to the average diet. They receive the majority of their B 17 from the many servings of apricot seeds that they eat each day.

The secret of the apricot kernels and B 17 lies in the fact they contain glycoside, a non-toxic form of cyanide, surrounded by sugar molecules. We know cancer cells love sugar, so they gobble up the amygdalin, (B 17).

Healthy cells contain an enzyme called Rhodanase that neutralizes the cyanide in B 17. But lo and behold, cancer cells do not have that Rhodanase enzyme that neutralizes the cyanide. Instead, they have another type of enzyme that creates a chemical reaction that creates the poisonous version of cyanide and kills the cancer cell. Poof! Another beautiful example of selective toxicity, very similar to blood root.

Studies have shown that amygdalin stops the production[275] of new blood vessels, suppresses inflammatory responses[276], and induces apoptosis or cell death[277] in various types of cancers.

---

[275] http://www.ncbi.nlm.nih.gov/pubmed/22771646
[276] http://www.ncbi.nlm.nih.gov/pubmed/21756879
[277] http://www.ncbi.nlm.nih.gov/pubmed/16880611

Apricot kernels contain the highest amounts of nitrilosides but here is a list of foods that are a rich source of this amazing phyto-nutrient:

- Apple seeds
- Millet
- Fava beans
- Wild blackberries
- Wild crabapples
- Choke cherries

I purchase my apricot kernels from Apricot Power[278] and keep a bag on my desk. I munch on them throughout the day and also include them in my smoothies. I grind them and sprinkle them on my salads and veggies.

It is recommended that you gradually introduce these potent seeds to your diet. Introducing them too fast can cause nausea. Start with 1 per hour, gradually increasing. A good rule of thumb is about 1 apricot kernel for every 10 pounds of body weight. So if you weigh 150 pounds, then you would consume 15 per day, spread out throughout the day. For serious health issues, some have taken as many as 25 - 40 per day.

Laetrile has been used successfully for over 50 years in many cancer clinics outside the United States in the form of IVs as well as in supplement form. One of these clinics is the well-known cancer treatment center in Mexico called the Oasis of Hope[279]. Their survival rate is quite impressive considering many people go there as a last resort, after they have been sent home to die from failed chemo and radiation.

BROCCOLI SPROUTS

Now who would have thought that little broccoli sprouts would be classified as a Tumor Terminator? You will be amazed to learn about all the research that supports the effectiveness of the phyto-

---

[278] http://www.apricotpower.com/#oid=80_1

[279] http://www.oasisofhope.com/

compounds in broccoli sprouts. The key ingredient that we are interested in is called Sulforaphane.

Although raw cruciferous vegetables contain Sulforaphane, the highest form is found in the broccoli sprout, containing 20-50 times more Sulforaphane than the mature vegetable.

You can view Sulforaphane as a messenger or 'signaling molecule' that activates around 200 genetic switches within the cell. Sometimes these switches are turned off because they are 'sleeping' or turned off because of toxicity and foreign chemicals.

Sulforaphane in broccoli sprouts plays a major role in stimulating the production of glutathione, a very powerful anti-oxidant that is produced inside the cell. As long as there is plenty of glutathione in your cells, then your cells are protected from damaging free radicals and toxins.

Another powerful role that Sulforaphane plays in your healing journey is that it turns on detoxification enzymes that help neutralize toxic molecules that could damage your cells.

In Chapter 1, you learned that your DNA is NOT your destiny because of little switches that are on your genes that can be turned off or on with your food choices. In following that train of thought, we could say that Sulforaphane 'talks to your DNA' by influencing how your DNA expresses itself through the genetic patterns. Changes in the expression of our genes can have a powerful effect on your overall health.

This is just a sample of some of the research studies conducted on Sulforaphane and its effect on Breast Cancer:

- Inhibits growth of Breast Cancer cells.[280]
- Decreases Breast Cancer cell migration and tumor formation.[281]
- Prevents Breast Cancer stem cell formation.[282]

---

[280] http://www.ncbi.nlm.nih.gov/pubmed/24289589
[281] http://www.ncbi.nlm.nih.gov/pubmed/24002734

- Impacts cancer prevention.[283]
- Induces Breast Cancer cell death.[284]
- Potent inhibitor of Breast Cancer.[285]
- Suppresses the growth and metastasis of Breast Cancer.[286]
- Decreases inflammatory effects of chemical toxins.[287]
- Enhances Natural Killer Cell Activity and Immune function.[288]

There are over 60 research articles on Sulforaphane and its effect on cancer. How exciting is that?

Broccoli sprouts were part of my regime in my healing journey and I still take them to this day. As with all the products that I personally use and recommend, I dug deep and found the best source of broccoli sprouts being manufactured in Australia. I spoke with Dr. Christine Houghton[289], the Chief Scientific Officer of the company, in order to understand what made their product better than others.

The difference was the superior strain of broccoli seed and the purity of specialized technology for growing the sprouts. The sprouts are harvested at their peak and dried at low temperatures so as to not affect the enzymes that create the Sulforaphane.

1 teaspoon powder of Enduracell Broccoli Sprout Powder is equivalent to 1⅓ pounds of broccoli and yields 60 mg. of Sulforaphane. While I was on my healing journey, I would add 1 teaspoon of broccoli powder to about 4 ounces of water and a few drops of stevia to sweeten the grassy taste, ☺, and did that twice per day. Since I am still very proactive with prevention, I enjoy the sprouts powder once per day.

---

282 http://www.ncbi.nlm.nih.gov/pubmed/23752191
283 http://www.ncbi.nlm.nih.gov/pubmed/23657153
284 http://www.ncbi.nlm.nih.gov/pubmed/22975350
285 http://www.ncbi.nlm.nih.gov/pubmed/23389114
286 http://www.ncbi.nlm.nih.gov/pubmed/21617865
287 http://www.ncbi.nlm.nih.gov/pubmed/16905640
288 http://www.ncbi.nlm.nih.gov/pubmed/17723168
289 http://www.cell-logic.com/index.php?option=com_content&task=view&id=13&Itemid=27

The great news is that Enduracell products are now available in the United States and through my store.[290]

CURCUMIN

Curcumin is derived from the roots of the turmeric, a very well-known Indian spice. There is a wealth of data supporting the power of curcumin in preventing and healing a wide range of diseases, from cancer to arthritic conditions to cardio vascular disease. One of the most important aspects of curcumin is being able to nip disease in the bud by down-regulating a gene switch that promotes chronic inflammation.[291]

The United States National Library of Medicine has over 200 studies specifically on the effectiveness of curcumin and Breast Cancer.

Here are a few benefits of incorporating curcumin in your healing journey:

- Decreases the survival rate of Breast Cancer cells.[292]
- Has anti-cancer properties and prevents tumor development.[293]
- Inhibits the spread and proliferation of Breast Cancer cells.[294]
- Induces apoptosis and cell suicide in Breast Cancer cells.[295]
- Reduces side effects of chemotherapy and improves the benefits of the drug.[296]
- Could provide an improved survival rate with triple negative Breast Cancer.[297]

---

[290] http://breastcancerconquerorshop.com/product/broccoli-sprout-powder/
[291] http://www.ncbi.nlm.nih.gov/pubmed/17569208
[292] http://www.ncbi.nlm.nih.gov/pubmed/21713389
[293] http://www.ncbi.nlm.nih.gov/pubmed/19908170
[294] http://www.ncbi.nlm.nih.gov/pubmed/21713389
[295] http://www.ncbi.nlm.nih.gov/pubmed/20646066
[296] http://www.ncbi.nlm.nih.gov/pubmed/19703194
[297] http://www.ncbi.nlm.nih.gov/pubmed/19809577

- Possible lead compound that would be helpful against multi-drug resistant Breast Cancer.[298]
- Pesticides have an estrogen effect on breast cells and stimulate Breast Cancer development. Curcumin has been found to have an inhibitory effect on the development of this type of cancer.[299]

However, not all curcumin supplements are created equally. Although curcumin has an impressive array of benefits, poor absorption through the digestive system has limited its bio-availability. Scientific formulations of curcumin have been able to elevate the bio-availability of curcumin up to 7 times higher than conventional curcumin.[300]

GcMAF

Although I have not used this particular product, I have read so much about it and its ability to destroy cancer cells that I felt compelled to share the information with you.

GcMAF is a Vitamin D binding protein that activates and stimulates macrophages, a type of white blood cell that eats Breast Cancer cells or any cancer cell for that matter.[301] Another great reason to make sure your Vitamin D3 levels are optimal!

GcMAF also prevents Breast Cancer cells from spreading and creating their own blood flow (angiogenesis).[302]

Dr. Nobuto Yamamoto[303], a research biochemist, discovered GcMAF and has spent over 20 years studying the tumoricidal effects of macrophages, the principle soldiers of your Immune System. Macrophages are like big Mack trucks compared to tiny cancer cells. They have long arms that engulf and surround the defective cells, then eat it, and digest it.

---

298 http://www.ncbi.nlm.nih.gov/pubmed/19250217
299 http://www.ncbi.nlm.nih.gov/pubmed/9168916
300 https://www.levitamins.com/54692/ProductDetails?item=00407
301 http://www.ncbi.nlm.nih.gov/pubmed/23857228
302 http://www.ncbi.nlm.nih.gov/pubmed/22213287
303 http://gcmaf.timsmithmd.com/book/chapter/65/

However, cancer cells have their own defense weapons against the Immune System. Cancer cells produce an enzyme called Nagalase that blocks GcMAF production, which puts the macrophages to sleep. Without the activation of GcMAF, cancer cells (and viruses and HIV) grow without restraint.

Enter Dr. Yamamoto's research.

Three specific studies showed that very small weekly doses of injectable GcMAF cured early metastatic Breast, Prostate, and Colon cancers 100% of the time in non-anemic patients!

And this was after the Big 3 Therapies of chemo, radiation, and surgery had failed.

To learn more about this amazing and promising therapy, read Dr. Tim Smith's *GcMAF Book*.[304] It is easy to read, and he has it posted on line for FREE! What a gift.

Where does one purchase GcMAF? First Immune[305] seems to be a reputable company but do your research and compare pricing and support.

HAELAN 951 – FERMENTED SOY

My personal use of this product takes me way back to the mid-90s when I was dealing with a serious health challenge. I drank several cases of Haelan along with other herbal tinctures. Over a period of time, my health dramatically improved.

I continued to recommend Haelan to many patients who had a deficient Immune System and saw remarkable results. After 'retiring' from my brick and mortar practice, I lost touch with Haelan for a few years. But as serendipitous events occur, it came back around into my life. It is now a part of my daily prevention plan.

So what exactly is Haelan? It is a very concentrated fermented, organic, non GMO soy beverage that was developed in China in the early 1980s as a nutritional supplement to be used in hospitals. It has

---

304 http://gcmaf.timsmithmd.com/
305 http://www.gcmaf.eu/

several patents on the manufacturing process and technology that makes Haelan a very unique soy product.

One 8 ounce bottle of Haelan contains 25 pounds of soy, indicating the potency and the concentration of the product. The phyto-chemical content in soybeans can vary, depending on the condition of the soil and when the beans are picked. Spectral analysis of soy products versus Haelan indicate a much greater concentration of isoflavones and genistein in Haelan 951.[306]

Here are some of the benefits of adding Haelan to your prevention or healing journey. In a nutshell, Haelan is a multi-faceted cancer killer.[307]

- Stops the production of the formation of new blood vessels (angiogenesis) that feed tumors.
- Inhibits development of Breast Cancer tumors.[308]
- Induces Apoptosis which means it causes cancer cells to self-destruct.[309]
- Increases the cancer killing effect of Natural Killer cells.
- Increases the macrophage activity. These are cells that gobble up and eat cancer cells.
- Increases the healthier estrogen (2-hydroxyestrone) levels and helps to metabolize the carcinogenic estrogens (4 and 16 hydroxyestrogens).[310]
- Blocks and protects estrogen receptor sites from more aggressive and dangerous estrogens.
- Lowers your Breast Cancer risk.[311]
- Stimulation of tumor suppressor genes.[312]

---

306 http://www.thrivinghealthandwellness.com/uploads/9100_-_Townsend_Ltr_-_Not_All_Soy_Products_are_Created_Equal_-_WHW.pdf

307 http://weeksmd.com/2011/08/haelan-multi-faceted-cancer-killer/

308 http://www.ncbi.nlm.nih.gov/pubmed/22954488

309 http://www.ncbi.nlm.nih.gov/pubmed/12588701

310 http://www.thrivinghealthandwellness.com/uploads/9150_-Townsend__Ltr_AugSept_2010_The_Mgmt_of_Estrogens_etc.pdf

311 http://www.ncbi.nlm.nih.gov/pubmed/23635365

312 http://www.ncbi.nlm.nih.gov/pubmed/11496322

- Converts cancer stem cells to normal healthy stem cells.[313]

Sound too good to be true? This formula was created by Chinese Medical Doctors and nutritionists to support the healing process of their hospitalized patients. Once they saw the miraculous results with their patients, this formula was shared with other doctors around the world.

You can order Haelan through my on-line store. If you have any questions about how you may benefit from Haelan 951, contact me through my web site.[314]

HEMP OIL AND CBD

Although the hemp plant has a reputation as a recreational 'drug', it contains medicinal qualities that have a positive impact on healing cancer. There are many components to the hemp plant but the 2 most commonly known ingredients are THC and CBD. THC is what gives you the sensation of feeling 'high and giddy' whereas the CBD (cannabidiol) is what has the most powerful anti-cancer properties.

Research scientists in San Francisco compiled data showing that CBD may actually heal cancer.[315] They found that CBD has a specific effect on metastatic cancer cells and aggressive tumor cells.

Through many detailed experiments, CBD was found to:[316]

- Trigger cell death
- Stopped cancer cells from dividing
- Prevented new blood vessels that feed tumors to grow
- Stopped cancer cells from invading neighboring tissue

Metastasis or spread of Breast Cancer is a major challenge for many women. CBD offers hope as a potential anti-metastatic therapy[317].

---

313 http://weeksmd.com/2011/08/converting-cancer-stem-cells-to-normal-stem-cells-haelan-led-the-way-science-catches-up/

314 http://breastcancerconqueror.com/about-dr-v/contact/

315 http://blogs.ocweekly.com/navelgazing/2013/04/bay_area_researchers_claim_can.php

316 http://www.ncbi.nlm.nih.gov/pubmed/22555283

317 http://www.ncbi.nlm.nih.gov/pubmed/22963825

CBD caused programmed cell death[318] in Breast Cancer cells and significantly reduced tumor[319] cell mass.

According to Molecular Cancer Therapy[320], CBD represents the first NON-TOXIC exogenous agent that can significantly decrease the expression in metastatic Breast Cancer cells and down-regulate tumor aggressiveness.

Estrogen overload from environmental chemicals and poor estrogen metabolism is responsible for many aggressive Breast Cancers. However, CBD has shown anti-estrogenic[321] properties, without any toxic side effects similar to aromatase inhibiting drugs like Tamoxifen. I have used hemp oil internally and topically as part of my healing protocol and enjoyed many of the benefits. I encourage you to take a look at the Rick Simpson Protocol[322], a Canadian who has helped many sick people get well and become cancer-free with the use of hemp oil.

Real Scientific Hemp Oil (RSHO) is derived from federally-legal industrial hemp plant. Their unique hemp cultivars, combined with their proprietary technology, produces the highest quality CBD-rich hemp in the world.

Become familiar with the legalities in your state, province, or country before attempting to use this.

---

318 http://www.ncbi.nlm.nih.gov/pubmed/21566064
319 http://www.ncbi.nlm.nih.gov/pubmed/20859676
320 http://www.ncbi.nlm.nih.gov/pubmed/18025276
321 http://www.ncbi.nlm.nih.gov/pubmed/16392670
322 http://ascendingstarseed.wordpress.com/2013/11/07/spain-study-confirms-hemp-oil-cures-cancer-without-side-effects/

SALICINIUM

I became familiar with this protocol after reading Suzanne Somers' book, *Knockout, Interviews with Doctors That Are Curing Cancer*.[323] This is an excellent book to help you build confidence in groundbreaking, non-toxic cancer curing protocols. Suzanne interviews some of today's forward thinking Medical Doctors that are using proven and innovative cancer treatments to heal cancer.

In Chapter 9 of the book, Dr. James Forsythe, a board certified homeopath and oncologist, discusses the success rates he had with Stage IV Breast and Prostate Cancer patients.

In a study of 350 patients using his protocol with Salicinium, also known as Orasal, and Poly MVA, he showed an 85% success rate after 4 years.

HST Global, a publicly held biotechnology and wellness company, has the rights to pre-clinical outcome based study using Salicinium. They found a 79% success rate in 250 women with Stage IV Breast Cancers at 33 months.[324]

So how does Salicinium work? Let's go back to cancer cell physiology 101.

Remember that cancer cells love sugar because they use it in a fermentation process that keeps them alive. Unlike healthy cells, they do not 'breathe' oxygen, but they use sugar to keep multiplying. When cancer cells multiply and divide, they produce an enzyme that cloaks or hides the cancer cells from our Immune System. (Remember the story of the Mack-truck macrophages that eat cancer cells?)

Salicinium can be ingested orally or given in an IV solution. Since Salicinium is a glycome, or sugar based molecule (are you seeing the patterns with natural medicine and sugar molecules?), the cancer

---

[323] http://www.suzannesomers.com/products/knockout-interviews-with-doctors-who-are-curing-cancer-and-how-to-prevent-getting-it-in-the-first-place-autographed

[324] http://www.reuters.com/article/2008/07/29/idUS156541+29-Jul-2008+BW20080729

cells gobble it up. Once this glycome is inside the cancer cell, it interrupts the fermentation and stops the production of the enzyme that cloaks or hides the cancer cell from the Immune System.

According to HST Global, this plant based natural substance alters malignant cell fermentation, blocks cell division, and weakens the cancer cell so they cannot withstand the attack from the Immune System.[325]

Here are a few key points about Salicinium:

- It is non-toxic and has no side effects
- It targets only cancer cells
- It can be used orally or in IV form
- It can be used in conjunction with other medical therapies
- It works best when the body is properly alkalized and has an abundance of healthy probiotics in the gut to enhance the Immune System

This powerful herbal therapy holds promise for many women that are on a healing journey. If you are very challenged with your health, consider doing the IV protocol under the supervision of a licensed health care professional.

You can learn more about this protocol by visiting my website.[326]

POLY MVA

Poly MVA is a unique, liquid formulation of minerals, vitamins, and amino acids that support cellular energy and metabolism. Dr. John Forsythe used Poly MVA in conjunction with Salicinium.

Poly MVA supports normal energy production of ATP by increasing oxygen and oxygen pathways inside the cell. Since we know that cancer cells do not like oxygen and 'breathe' with sugar fermentation, Poly MVA nutrients interfere with the cancer cells' metabolism.

---

325 http://www.reuters.com/article/2008/07/29/idUS156541+29-Jul-2008+BW20080729

326 http://breastcancerconquerorshop.com/product-category/perfect-balance/

It supports the liver in removing toxic substances from the body, and it works as a powerful anti-oxidant. As with any other protocol, get educated, make informed decisions, and find professional help to guide you through this process.

In this article[327], I discuss the Poly MVA protocol and recommended dosage.

You can find very encouraging testimonials about Poly MVA as well as survivor stories through this web site.[328]

SPIRULINA

You may wonder why I have classified Spirulina, fresh water algae, as a Tumor Terminator. From a nutritional point of view, Spirulina is a high protein food that is about 60% protein. It is loaded with healthy Omega 3s like GLA, EPA, DHA, and ALA. It has 300% more calcium than dairy products and 3900% more beta carotene than carrots.

One half teaspoon of Spirulina has more anti-oxidant and anti-inflammatory power than 5 servings of vegetables.[329]

Here are a few examples of the power of Spirulina:

- It enhances your Immune System.[330]
- It can potentially prevent malignancy.[331]
- It has many anti-cancer properties and induces cancer cell death.[332]
- Reduced incidence of breast tumors from 87% to 13% in laboratory animals.[333]
- Reduced expression of proteins that increase cellular proliferation.[334]

---

[327] http://breastcancerconqueror.com/have-you-heard-of-poly-mva/
[328] http://www.polymvasurvivors.com/
[329] http://breastcancerconqueror.com/spirulina-a-powerful-anti-cancer-super-food/
[330] http://www.ncbi.nlm.nih.gov/pubmed/23743830
[331] http://www.ncbi.nlm.nih.gov/pubmed/23633807
[332] http://www.ncbi.nlm.nih.gov/pubmed/23134462
[333] http://www.ncbi.nlm.nih.gov/pubmed/24269837

- Induced Breast Cancer cell death in 48 hours.[335]

Anti-cancer effects have been noted (Md Saad et al., 2006) when 150 mgs. per pound of body weight of Spirulina were ingested. For example, a 200 pound person would ingest 6 teaspoons per day while a smaller framed woman would do well to add 3-4 teaspoons of Spirulina to her diet. This can be accomplished by adding Spirulina to your smoothies or ingesting it in capsule form.[336]

I have now given you ample evidence of the power of natural medicine and its effect on cancer. I trust this will encourage you and give you confidence in herbal and natural 'tumor terminators'. Consult with your health care provider and decide what may work best for you.

In any protocol, it is important to weaken cancer cells, but it is just as important to boost the power of your Immune System. Next, I will discuss specific herbs and natural substances that boost your Immune System.

BODY BUILDERS THAT BOOST YOUR IMMUNE SYSTEM

Your Immune System is an intricate system with many components. According to the National Institute of Health, your immune system is a network of cells, tissues, and organs that work together against any foreign invaders. The secret to the success of the Immune System is its communication system. Remember how the cancer cells sent out enzymes that cloaked themselves from the Immune System and even put the Mack-truck macrophages to sleep?

This is why it is so important to make sure your Immune System is working at full capacity. If you have developed cancer, it is an indication that your immunity was tired and your body was toxic. Mother Nature has blessed us with so many amazing gifts in the form of powerful immune boosters.

---

334 http://www.ncbi.nlm.nih.gov/pubmed/24269837

335 http://www.ncbi.nlm.nih.gov/pubmed/24269837

336 http://breastcancerconquerorshop.com/product/cancer-x-spirulina-1-lb-powder/

BETA GLUCANS

Beta Glucans are poly saccharides (complex sugar molecules) that are extracted from medicinal mushrooms. Medicinal mushrooms have been used for thousands of years across the globe. There is an abundance of research concerning the effect of Beta Glucans on the Immune System.[337] They increase the activity of the Mack Truck macrophages, inhibit the growth of tumor cells, and weaken Breast Cancer genes.

Beta Glucans stimulate immunity by activation of macrophages and can increase the benefits of therapies in women with advanced Breast Cancer.[338]

As with any product, there is the 'real deal' and the 'wannabes'. Beta 1, 3 D Glucan by Transfer Point, Inc. is the real deal.[339] They have numerous independent laboratory studies that prove that not all Glucans are created equal and that many of the other commercial Glucans exhibit very low immune activity. Bill Henderson, a wise and gentle cancer coach, has recommended this product for years with great success.[340] Beta Glucans are a part of my daily maintenance plan.

To order Beta 1, 3 D Glucan, simply head to my store.[341]

CHAGA

Chaga is a medicinal mushroom that grows in the wild and is hand harvested. It has a similar effect on the Immune System as the 1, 3 Beta Glucans since it has 30% beta glucans by weight. I personally used Chaga extract[342] and to this day, enjoy drinking it as a tea[343], but you can also take it in capsule form. The extract has been found to be more potent than eating the whole mushroom.

---

337 http://www.ncbi.nlm.nih.gov/pubmed/19053851
338 http://www.ncbi.nlm.nih.gov/pubmed/17161824
339 http://www.transferpoint.com/aboutus.asp
340 http://www.beating-cancer-gently.com/
341 http://breastcancerconquerorshop.com/product/beta-13-d-glucan/
342 http://breastcancerconquerorshop.com/product/chaga-750-ct/
343 http://breastcancerconquerorshop.com/product/chaga-tea-1lb/

Chaga extracts have demonstrated strong anti-bacterial effects as well as anti-proliferative effects on Breast Cancer cells.[344] Results of studies suggest that Chaga extracts could be used as a natural anti-cancer ingredient.[345]

ESSIAC TEA

Rene Caisse was a Canadian nurse who lived in northern Ontario in the 1920s. She was introduced to a combination of herbs that showed promise in regressing cancer and named the tea Essiac, which is her name spelled backwards.

As she began sharing her tea with those searching for improved health, she was soon treating 300-600 cancer patients per week. She continued serving humanity for over 8 years, until the Canadian government shut down her clinic.

There were 8 medical doctors that witnessed hundreds of reversals in cancer patients and each wrote an affidavit to that effect.

Rene was quoted as saying, "Chemotherapy should be a criminal offense. Essiac Tea is harmless."

I could not agree with her more! Why is it that gross poisoning and mutilation through chemotherapy is regarded as 'safe science' while beneficial and harmless natural medicines are labeled quackery?

There are 4 main ingredients in true Essiac Tea:

- Burdock Root
- Sheep Sorrel
- Slippery Elm
- Turkey Rhubarb Root

In combination, these stimulate the Immune System, purify the blood, reduce inflammation, and have anti-cancer properties. The

---

[344] http://www.ncbi.nlm.nih.gov/pubmed/24380885
[345] http://www.ncbi.nlm.nih.gov/pubmed/20607061

Alternative Cancer Care website[346] has many research studies about the power of Essiac Tea.

The best source for learning more about the real Essiac Tea is from Health Freedom Network.[347]

HERBAL SUPPORT AND HOMEOPATHY

There are many herbs that have shown tremendous effects on cancer. The tinctures that I am most familiar with are from Bio-Active Nutritionals.[348] I have personally and professionally used these herbs for over 20 years:

Artemesia, also known as wormwood, has been shown to inhibit growth of Breast Cancer cells and has promising anti-cancer properties.[349]

Pau D'arco, also known as taheebo, has anti-proliferative effects on Breast Cancer cells and promotes apoptosis (cancer cell death).[350]

Una de Gato extracts, also known as cat's claw, have a direct anti-proliferative effect on Breast Cancer cells and possess anti-inflammatory properties.[351] Research scientists believe that it is a promising agent in the treatment of Breast Cancer and human sarcoma.[352]

Burdock has concentrations of lignans that have exhibited anti-cancer properties in animal models. It suppresses the growth of various cancers, including Breast Cancer.[353]

Tinctures are very easy to take since you simply add them to your drinking water and sip on them all day. These tinctures are available in my store and can be drop shipped to your home.

---

[346] http://www.alternative-cancer-care.com/essiac-tea-and-cancer.html
[347] http://www.healthfreedom.info/Cancer%20Essiac.htm
[348] http://breastcancerconquerorshop.com/product-category/homeopathics/
[349] http://www.ncbi.nlm.nih.gov/pubmed/22185819
[350] http://www.ncbi.nlm.nih.gov/pubmed/?term=pau+d%27arco++breast+cancer
[351] http://www.ncbi.nlm.nih.gov/pubmed/?term=una+de+gato+breast+cancer
[352] http://www.ncbi.nlm.nih.gov/pubmed/19724995
[353] http://www.ncbi.nlm.nih.gov/pubmed/18288407

Homeopathy is a system of medicine which involves dosing with highly diluted substances.[354] The theory is based on the model of 'like cures like' which means when a substance causes certain symptoms in large doses, it can relieve the symptoms in extremely minute, diluted doses. Rather than change the chemistry of the body, homeopathy affects the body energetically.

I have used homeopathy extensively for many years and have found it to be a beneficial adjunct to any protocol.

IP 6

IP 6 is inositol hexophosphate or phytic acid. It is a molecule of inositol (a B vitamin) and 6 molecules of phosphorus. IP 6 is found in dried beans, nuts, seeds, and rice. Dr. Abdul Shamsuddin, Ph.D., a Professor of Pathology at the University of Maryland School of Medicine, began his research on cancer in the 1970s.[355] He discovered that this particular plant compound had the ability to control the rate of abnormal cell division and boost Natural Killer cell activity.

But the most amazing discovery was that IP 6 had the ability to directly affect the cancer cell's metabolism of sugar. ***Research papers have shown that IP 6 inhibited Breast Cancer[356] cell growth by 50% and is effective for cancer prevention.[357]***

It may be used safely as an adjunctive therapy in ameliorating the side effects of chemotherapy.[358] The administration of phytic acid reversed the proliferative effects of cancer a cancer-causing chemical.[359]

If you get tired of swallowing pills, IP 6 can also be purchased in sugar-free powdered form.[360]

---

354 http://www.homeopathy-soh.org/about-homeopathy/what-is-homeopathy/
355 http://ip6gold.com/dr-shamsuddin/
356 http://www.ncbi.nlm.nih.gov/pubmed/22655458
357 http://www.ncbi.nlm.nih.gov/pubmed/21489580
358 http://www.ncbi.nlm.nih.gov/pubmed/20152024
359 http://www.ncbi.nlm.nih.gov/pubmed/16969125
360 http://breastcancerconquerorshop.com/product-category/essential-1-let-food-be-your-medicine/

PROBIOTICS

Probiotics are an essential part of boosting your Immune System. The general term probiotic literally means 'for life or supporting life'. Your intestines have over 500 different strains of bacteria which support digestion, the Immune System, and even produce certain vitamins, such as Vitamin Bs and Vitamin K. This army of bacteria also creates a line of defense against any unhealthy invaders. ***It has been said that 70% of your Immune System is in your gut; thus, a healthy gut equals a healthy Immune System.***

Aside from assisting in digestion, increasing number of studies have demonstrated many benefits of healthy bacterial strains when it comes to Breast Cancer:

- Reduction of cancer promoting enzymes.[361]
- Consumption of probiotics improved the production of Immune modulators.[362]
- Reduces the effects of chemotherapy induced diarrhea.[363]
- Delayed breast tumor growth in animal studies.[364]
- Probiotics are a potential agent in the prevention of Breast Cancer prevention, treatment and management.[365]
- Stimulates anti-tumor immunity in Breast Cancer models.[366]
- Significantly impact and Inhibit cancer progression.[367]

Daily supplementation with a solid, healthy strain of probiotics is extremely important for cancer prevention and for supporting the healing process. Fermented, raw vegetables and cultured milks (goat, coconut, raw, grass fed cow) are also a great source.

---

[361] http://www.ncbi.nlm.nih.gov/pubmed/18461293
[362] http://www.ncbi.nlm.nih.gov/pubmed/20193099
[363] http://www.ncbi.nlm.nih.gov/pubmed/19423769
[364] http://www.ncbi.nlm.nih.gov/pubmed/20550747
[365] http://www.ncbi.nlm.nih.gov/pubmed/22201894
[366] http://www.ncbi.nlm.nih.gov/pubmed/22711009
[367] http://www.ncbi.nlm.nih.gov/pubmed/24382758

NOURISHING NUTRIENTS THAT SUPPORT THE HEALING PROCESS

There are many specific nutrients that have strong anti-oxidant and anti-cancer effects. I will share the ones that I have found to be most effective, based on scientific research and personal and professional experience. In my opinion, these various nutrients may support your body as it endeavors to find balance and strength. Organic and raw food is always the best source of nutrients but when your body needs extra fuel to overcome stress and immune deficiencies, supplementation with some of these nutrients may prove helpful for you.

DIM AND I3C

Unfortunately, the word estrogen creates fear in most women. Estrogen has been given a bad rap because it is often associated with Breast Cancer. Estrogen is your friend and ally and not your foe.

As discussed in Chapter 3, there is now a new class of estrogens that add a burden to the body - xeno-estrogens. If estrogen is not metabolized properly because of a toxic liver and/or poor methylation then the harmful, aggressive estrogen will accumulate in the body.

There are certain compounds found in cruciferous vegetables, namely DIM and I3C, that help convert 'stronger' estrogens into benign and protective estrogens such as 2 -hydroxyestrone. Here are some of the reasons for including DIM and I3C in your healing or prevention protocol.

- Reduces your Breast Cancer risk.[368]
- Prevents the development of estrogen-enhanced cancers such as Breast, Cervical and Endometrial cancers.[369]
- DIM has the potential as an anti-metastatic agent for Breast Cancer.[370]

---

[368] http://www.ncbi.nlm.nih.gov/pubmed/22877795
[369] http://www.ncbi.nlm.nih.gov/pubmed/12840226
[370] http://www.ncbi.nlm.nih.gov/pubmed/19864400

- Inhibits the development of breast tumors by preventing the growth of new blood vessels (angiogenesis).[371]
- DIM down-regulates or weakens the protein surviving that keeps cancer cells from dying and thus encourages cancer cells to self-destruct.[372]
- I3C binds or blocks the estrogen receptor (ER alpha) that is activated by estrogen; thus, having an anti-tumor effect.[373]

You would have to eat 4-6 pounds of broccoli and cabbage in order to create 100 - 200 mg. of DIM. Supplementing with specific, clean formulas will support a healthy estrogen metabolism so you do not have to fear estrogen ever again.[374]

GLUTATHIONE

Glutathione is what we call a primary anti-oxidant because it is extremely potent and powerful. Glutathione is produced inside a healthy, well-nourished cell and is needed in order for other anti-oxidants to be properly utilized. It is also very important in detoxification pathways and immune system activity.

The bad news is that stress, toxins, pollution, aging, radiation, and infections deplete our glutathione reserves.

There are mixed theories about glutathione supplementation. Some advocates argue that glutathione can be taken orally and is not digested in the stomach. Others say that since glutathione is protein-based, it is impossible for glutathione to be ingested orally without being digested and the only way to increase glutathione in your body is by eating specific super-foods.

Personally, I tend to lean towards the super-food theory. If you can get it from nature instead of a pill, I believe that ALL the co-factors necessary to stimulate the production of it will be there.

---

[371] http://www.ncbi.nlm.nih.gov/pubmed/15661811
[372] http://www.ncbi.nlm.nih.gov/pubmed/16651453
[373] http://www.ncbi.nlm.nih.gov/pubmed/16488130
[374] http://breastcancerconquerorshop.com/product/dim-i3c-healthy-estrogen-support/

Here are the best ways to increase your glutathione production:

- Minimize and reduce your mental and physical stress since it depletes your glutathione reserves.
- Curcumin increases glutathione levels.[375]
- Eat plenty of organic sulfur-containing vegetables such as garlic and onions. Cruciferous vegetables, avocados, and parsley improve glutathione production.
- Raw, organic, hormone free whey[376] protein contains the highest levels of glutathione precursors that help improve glutathione production. Whey protein increases intracellular glutathione by 64%.[377]
- Regular exercise boosts glutathione production. Mover your body vigorously with burst training or brisk walk-runs at least 4 times per week for 20-30 minutes per day.
- Supportive liver herbs like Milk Thistle help boost glutathione levels.
- Broccoli sprouts have high levels of sulforaphane which stimulates glutathione production.[378] (Are you starting to see a pattern with the benefits of cruciferous vegetables?)
- Coffee enemas stimulate glutathione production.

FLAX SEEDS AND FLAX OIL

As always, I stand in awe of the healing power of yet another gift from Nature: flax seeds. Although flax is high in fiber, omega 3 fatty acids, vitamins, and minerals, its most beneficial component are *lignans.*

Lignans are chemical compounds that are classified as plant estrogens which act as strong anti-oxidants.

I recommend that you grind your flax seeds right before use. It keeps them fresher and more potent. ***Get into the habit of adding 5***

---

375 http://www.ncbi.nlm.nih.gov/pubmed/15650394
376 http://breastcancerconquerorshop.com/?s=whey&post_type=product
377 http://www.ncbi.nlm.nih.gov/pubmed/12537959
378 http://breastcancerconquerorshop.com/product/broccoli-sprout-powder/

teaspoons of freshly ground flax seeds to your smoothies, soups, or salads.

Flax seeds are a girl's best friend! Here's why:

- Premenopausal women who had a diet higher in plant lignans had a significantly reduced Breast Cancer risk.[379]
- Enterolactones from flax lignans have a very significant anti-metastatic effect.[380]
- Plant estrogens, such as flax seeds and (fermented) soy, may affect Breast Cancer progression in a similar fashion as Tamoxifen (but without all the side effects, of course.)[381]
- Activates programmed cell death in certain Breast Cancer cell lines.[382]
- Flax lignans have a strong protective effect on breast cells.[383]
- Increase the concentration of Sex Hormone Binding Globulin which lower estrogen levels.[384]

Adding flax to your diet can also improve post-menopausal depression and improve your brain function.

If you don't like adding flax to your diet, Barlean's offers a great product called Brevail.[385] Brevail is a concentrated and standardized product that is 100 fold higher in lignan concentration that most lignan bearing foods. This researched product was designed to increase lignan concentration to optimal levels. Adding a few capsules to your regime may prove very beneficial for your breast health.

IODINE

---

379 http://www.ncbi.nlm.nih.gov/pubmed/15221974
380 http://www.ncbi.nlm.nih.gov/pubmed/22842186
381 http://www.ncbi.nlm.nih.gov/pubmed/21097717
382 http://www.ncbi.nlm.nih.gov/pubmed/21520988
383 http://www.ncbi.nlm.nih.gov/pubmed/14687793
384 J Steroid Biochem 1987;27:1135-1144
385 http://breastcancerconquerorshop.com/product/brevail-2/

Discovering the connection with iodine and Breast Cancer was a huge AHA moment for me. I was equally as excited to learn that there was a simple home based urine test that could measure the extent of the deficiency.

Iodine is an essential trace element and nutrient that every cell in the body needs. Without it, many of our glandular tissues such as the thyroid, breast, uterus, ovaries, and prostate begin to develop nodules and cysts. The end result is fibrocystic breasts, polycystic ovaries, and uterine fibroids. ***According to Dr. David Brownstein's research, if these cysts are not corrected, the cells can develop hyperplasia (increased cell growth) which can lead to cancer.***[386]

There is a global iodine deficiency because of the commercialization of foods as well as the exposure to many bromides. Bromides, found in pesticides, flame retardants, food additives, and all our electronic devices, displace iodine in the cell, adding to the iodine deficiency problem. Fluorides and heavy metals also have a similar effect.

Iodine is needed for hormone production, such as thyroid hormones, sex hormones, insulin, growth hormones, etc. Interestingly, 1:7 women in the US are iodine deficient, while the incidence of Breast Cancer is 1:8. Unfortunately, when a woman shows up in a typical doctor's office with goiter, nodules, or thyroid symptoms, a prescription for toxic drugs will be prescribed, rather than prescribing an iodine-urine loading test to check for iodine deficiency.

Prescribing thyroid hormones to iodine deficient women could be a prescription for increasing the risk of Breast Cancer.[387]

There is more and more evidence linking Breast Cancer with thyroid disease.[388] Demographic studies indicate that countries that have a high intake of iodine, such as Japan and Iceland, also have a low incidence of Breast Cancer.[389]

---

386 http://www.drbrownstein.com/

387 http://www.newswithviews.com/Howenstine/james47.htm#_ftn10

388 http://www.ncbi.nlm.nih.gov/pubmed/?term=PMC314438

389 Finley JW, Bogardus, GM. Breast Cancer and Thyroid Disease Quart. Review Surg Obstet Gyn 17:139-147, 1960

Breast tissue has a trapping mechanism for iodine and actually competes for iodine. If there is low intake of iodine, then the thyroid and breast tissue suffer.

Iodine appears to be a requisite for healthy breast tissue.[390] If iodine is lacking, iodine deficient breasts are more susceptible to cancerous activity. Iodine is an anti-proliferative agent and contributes to the health of a normal breast.[391]

I believe that every woman who wants to prevent Breast Cancer, or is actually dealing with Breast Cancer, should have her iodine levels tested and supplement with Iodoral, (iodine and iodide formulation) accordingly.[392]

MAGNESIUM

As far back as the 1930s, doctors were writing about the benefits of magnesium for cancer prevention. In an enlightening article written by Professor Pierre Delbet in 1931 called *Take Magnesium and Escape Cancer*, he discusses how deficiency to magnesium predisposed people to cancer.

According to the National Institute of Health[393] and Office of Dietary Supplements, "Americans are not getting enough of the recommended amount of magnesium. Having enough body stores of magnesium may be protective against disorders such as cardiovascular disease and immune function."

Magnesium is involved in more than 300 enzymatic reactions in the body. It is needed for glutathione production, nerve and muscle function, DNA and RNA synthesis, synergy with iodine, and many other vital functions. Brazilian Medical and Biological Researches

---

[390] http://www.ncbi.nlm.nih.gov/pubmed/343535
[391] http://www.ncbi.nlm.nih.gov/pubmed/16025225
[392] http://breastcancerconquerorshop.com/product/urine-iodine-testing/
[393] http://ods.od.nih.gov/factsheets/Magnesium-HealthProfessional/#h3

have found that the incidence of low magnesium in critically ill cancer patients was very common.[394]

Magnesium deficiency[395] seems to be carcinogenic, while a high level of supplemented magnesium inhibits carcinogenesis. Drinking alcohol every day lowers your magnesium levels and increases your Breast Cancer risk by up to 30%.

Great sources of magnesium are green leafy vegetables like spinach and kale, nuts, seeds, and beans. As far as supplementation, I prefer magnesium glycinate[396] or a liposomal form[397] of magnesium. Magnesium is more easily absorbed and less irritating on the gut with these formulas.

Dr. Sircus, a Baking Soda and Magnesium advocate, suggests the use of Magnesium chloride flakes for baths or magnesium chloride gel to apply topically to the skin.[398] Topical magnesium therapy is very calming and is a great way to assist the body in detoxification.

If you are on a healing journey, magnesium therapy is a must.[399] Soak in pounds of magnesium chloride and rub the oil on the bottom of your feet and on your breasts.

MELATONIN – THE SMART KILLER

When it comes to Breast Cancer, melatonin could be a very helpful therapy to consider.

Let me begin by reminding you about the effect of EMFs on melatonin production. In Chapter 3, I discussed how melatonin actually put Breast Cancer cells to sleep but when the cells were exposed to EMFs,

---

394 http://www.scielo.br/scielo.php?script=sci_arttext&pid=S0100-879X2000001200007

395 http://www.ncbi.nlm.nih.gov/pubmed/3545048

396 http://breastcancerconquerorshop.com/product/optimal-magnesium/

397 http://breastcancerconquerorshop.com/product/liposomal-magnesium-original-flavor-10-oz/

398 http://drsircus.com/

399 http://www.ancient-minerals.com/magnesium-chloride/

melatonin had absolutely no effect in suppressing the growth of cancer cells.

If you live in a very isolated area and you do not have satellite and WIFI in your home, and don't use a cell phone, then perhaps supplementing with melatonin may not be as crucial for you. But I would venture to say that the average woman is exposed to too many EMFs.

In a meta-analysis, higher levels of morning urinary melatonin were associated with a decreased Breast Cancer risk.[400]

Melatonin behaves as a 'smart killer'[401] by keeping healthy cells alive while triggering suicide signals to cancer cells.

When it comes to Breast Cancer, melatonin is a powerful ally. It has an anti-estrogenic effect on estrogen receptors and reduces cell proliferation.[402] Melatonin levels are significantly associated with lower Breast Cancer risk in post-menopausal women.[403] It inhibits initiation[404] and growth of hormone-dependent tumors while at the same time inhibiting and preventing the growth[405] of new blood vessels that feed tumors.

Melatonin enhances DNA repair[406] capacity and even causes Breast Cancer cells to die![407]

Since melatonin production peaks in total darkness, make your bedroom a sleeping sanctuary. Remove all your electronic devices from your bedroom and never sleep with a cell phone or electric alarm clock by your head. Turn off all lights, even 'night lights' as this can affect your melatonin production.[408]

---

[400] http://www.ncbi.nlm.nih.gov/pubmed/24418683
[401] http://www.ncbi.nlm.nih.gov/pubmed/24032643
[402] http://www.ncbi.nlm.nih.gov/pubmed/19522736
[403] http://www.ncbi.nlm.nih.gov/pubmed/22237979
[404] http://www.ncbi.nlm.nih.gov/pubmed/21995112
[405] http://www.ncbi.nlm.nih.gov/pubmed/24416386
[406] http://www.ncbi.nlm.nih.gov/pubmed/23294620
[407] http://www.ncbi.nlm.nih.gov/pubmed/22335196
[408] http://jbr.sagepub.com/content/12/6/575.refs

The light emitted from cell phones, computers, hand held I pads, and televisions emit a light that reduces your melatonin production so prepare yourself for bed at least 1 hour before you get into bed by pulling away from all electronic devices.

Food sources that improve production of melatonin include nuts, seeds, Spirulina, and beans. Supplementing with tryptophan and making sure you have the building blocks for proper melatonin production is important. These include B6 and B3 (niacinamide.)

Life Extension[409] has many interesting research articles about melatonin and its effect on cancer. While optimal dosing has not been established when it comes to cancer patients, clinical studies have shown that 10-50 mgs. of melatonin have proven beneficial for cancer patients.

OMEGA 3 FATTY ACIDS

The industrialization of our food has caused an imbalance of our healthy oil intake. There are too may Omega 6s from plant oils that are used in fast foods and in food processing. Omega 3s from raw nuts and seeds as well from wild caught salmon are extremely important for breast health. ***Decreased Breast Cancer risk is associated with the intake of healthy, unsaturated, fatty acids while an intake of saturated fats and trans fats increases the Breast Cancer risk.***[410]

In a study involving over 880,000 participants, higher consumption of dietary marine PUFA (poly unsaturated fatty acids) was associated with a lower Breast Cancer risk.[411] Do you have a problem with dense, lumpy breasts? Higher intake of Omega 3s is associated with lower breast density, suggesting that it could be a strategy for Breast Cancer prevention.[412]

---

409 http://www.lef.org/magazine/mag2004/jan2004_report_melatonin_03.htm?source=search&key=melatonin%20and%20cancer

410 http://www.ncbi.nlm.nih.gov/pubmed/23137008

411 http://www.ncbi.nlm.nih.gov/pubmed/23814120

412 http://www.ncbi.nlm.nih.gov/pubmed/24402865

Omega 3s actually shift the estrogen signaling to inhibit Breast Cancer cell growth![413] Data from a study done in 2013 indicates that Omega 3s keep Breast Cancer cells from spreading and growing by inducing cell death![414]

If you don't like the idea of eating fish or taking fish oils, walnuts decreased the growth rate of Breast Cancer by 80% and reduced the number of tumors on laboratory animals by 60%![415]

Flax seeds and flax oil are also a great source of Omega 3s so remember to add those freshly ground flax seeds to your smoothies and salads.

SELENIUM

Selenium is a trace mineral that is essential for over 2 dozen biochemical reactions involved in thyroid metabolism, reproduction, and protection from oxidative stress. There are various forms of selenium that act in different pathways; so, supplementing with the proper selenium is important. Life Extension has a complete form of selenium[416] that has all 3 forms of selenium plus added Vitamin E for better absorption:

- Sodium selenite
- L-selenomethionine
- Selenium-methyl L-selenocysteine

Selenium deficiency can pose a significant health risk, since selenium is needed to make the enzyme that stimulates glutathione production.

The best food sources of selenium include: Brazil nuts, sardines, chicken and turkey, and spinach. But even if you eat plenty of these foods, if you are being proactive with prevention or if you are on a healing journey, supplementing with the proper selenium is very important.

---

[413] http://www.ncbi.nlm.nih.gov/pubmed/23285198
[414] http://www.ncbi.nlm.nih.gov/pubmed/23168911
[415] http://www.ncbi.nlm.nih.gov/pubmed/24500939
[416] https://www.levitamins.com/54692/ProductDetails?item=01778

Selenium inhibits estrogen induced[417] Breast Cancer cells while the lack of selenium[418] may increase the risk for progression of Breast Cancer and metastasis. Selenium has been credited with having high anti-cancer properties and the ability to prevent metastasis.[419]

Poor survival rates are associated with low selenium levels.[420]

Scientists analyzed selenium levels in Breast Cancer tumors and discovered that tissue levels of selenium were lower in Breast Cancer compared to fibrotic cysts.

Since selenium inhibits carcinogenesis, they concluded that low tissue levels of selenium may be associated with the development of Breast Cancer.[421]

VITAMIN C

Vitamin C can be incorporated in your regime in many forms. You can take plain ascorbic acid, Ester C, liposomal C and if you have access to a physician that administers IV Vitamin C infusions, then you have that option as well. As much as 50 - 70 grams of Vitamin C can be supplied through IV on a daily basis.

According to the National Institute of Health, "Laboratory and animal studies using Vitamin C have shown that it slows the growth and spread of several types of cancer."[422] High doses of Vitamin C produce large amounts of hydrogen peroxide which kills off cancer cells.

The research behind Vitamin C is staggering. In a nutshell, it acts as a powerful anti-oxidant and anti-inflammatory agent.[423] It has been shown to inhibit the growth and spread of Breast Cancer cells.[424] In the Breast Cancer Pooling Project, over 12,000 Breast Cancer

---

[417] http://www.ncbi.nlm.nih.gov/pubmed/22975630
[418] http://www.ncbi.nlm.nih.gov/pubmed/23429470
[419] http://www.ncbi.nlm.nih.gov/pubmed/23613334
[420] http://www.ncbi.nlm.nih.gov/pubmed/23704933
[421] http://www.ncbi.nlm.nih.gov/pubmed/23959347
[422] http://www.cancer.gov/cancertopics/pdq/cam/highdosevitaminc/patient/page2
[423] http://www.ncbi.nlm.nih.gov/pubmed/22963460
[424] http://www.ncbi.nlm.nih.gov/pubmed/23175106

survivors from the United States and China were assessed.[425] The analysis indicated a decreased risk of death with the use of Vitamin C and other anti-oxidants.

Vitamin C has also had a very positive effect on improving the quality of life for women undergoing radiation and chemotherapy.[426] Symptoms such as nausea, fatigue, depression, sleep disorders, and dizziness were drastically improved.

In combination with Beta Glucans and resveratrol, Vitamin C suppressed the growth of breast and lung tumors.[427] This is an example of the beneficial effects of putting all of this into practice. You can feel confident that the correct program of supplementation will work synergistically to improve your health.

VITAMIN D

If you are not spending at least 1 hour per day in exposing most of your body to sunlight, you should consider supplementing with Vitamin D3. When I consult with women all over the globe, the daily dosage may vary from 1,000 to 50,000 I.U. s of Vitamin D3. How do you determine your proper dosage? Have your physician run some blood work to test your levels. If that is not possible, here is a simple finger-prick home test that you can do in the privacy of your home.[428]

Once you know how deficient you are, then you can supplement accordingly. Here is an important note about supplementing with Vitamin D. According to Dr. R. Bleue, when you take Vitamin D, you are creating an increased need for Vitamin K2. Vitamin K2 is manufactured in your intestinal tract, IF you have a healthy gut. However, it is recommended that you supplement with a formula that contains the proper ratios of K1, K2, and D3.[429]

---

[425] http://www.ncbi.nlm.nih.gov/pubmed/23660948
[426] http://www.ncbi.nlm.nih.gov/pubmed/22021693
[427] http://www.ncbi.nlm.nih.gov/pubmed/22213291
[428] http://breastcancerconquerorshop.com/product/vitamin-d-blood-drop-test/
[429] https://www.levitamins.com/54692/ProductDetails?item=01741

Now that we are clear on getting the proper dosage, how does Vitamin D3 affect Breast Cancer prevention and healing? ***There are over 500 studies on the benefits of Vitamin D and Breast Cancer on the United States National Library of Medicine's website.***[430]

Here are a few highlights:

- Promising preventative agent for Breast Cancer.[431]
- Higher circulating blood levels are associated with reduced risk of post-menopausal Breast Cancer.[432]
- Inhibits Breast Cancer cell growth.[433]
- Inhibits inflammatory factors associated with cancer.[434]
- Stimulates Mack Truck Macrophages to attack Breast Cancer cells.[435]
- Suppresses cancer cell migration.[436]
- Suppresses proteins that are required for survival of triple negative Breast Cancer cells.[437]

A large placebo-controlled study[438] on Vitamin D and cancer indicated that it decreased overall cancer risk by as much as 77%! The results of this study were so compelling that the Canadian Cancer Society began endorsing the use of Vitamin D as a cancer prevention therapy.

ZINC

Zinc is another mineral that is essential for a strong Immune System since it helps maintain the thymus gland. It stimulates the activity of

---

430 http://www.ncbi.nlm.nih.gov/pubmed/?term=vitamin+d3+breast+cancer
431 http://www.ncbi.nlm.nih.gov/pubmed/24244740
432 http://www.ncbi.nlm.nih.gov/pubmed/24438060
433 http://www.ncbi.nlm.nih.gov/pubmed/23700865
434 http://www.ncbi.nlm.nih.gov/pubmed/24023320
435 http://www.ncbi.nlm.nih.gov/pubmed/23857228
436 http://www.ncbi.nlm.nih.gov/pubmed/23584482
437 http://www.ncbi.nlm.nih.gov/pubmed/24239860
438 http://www.ncbi.nlm.nih.gov/pubmed?orig_cmd=Search&term=Am.+J.+Clin.+Nutr.%5BJour%5D+AND+2007%5Bpdat%5D+AND+Lappe+J%5Bauthor%5D

over 300 enzymatic reactions but is especially important for the production of SOD (superoxide dismutase), one of the most potent free radical scavengers in the body.

Zinc is very inexpensive and can easily be added to your protocol.[439] Zinc deficiency is prevalent worldwide. Zinc not only improves your immune function, but it acts as an anti-inflammatory agent. ***It also decreases the formation of new blood vessels that feed tumors while increasing cancer cell death!***[440]

The cleanest food sources of zinc are grass fed clean meats, beans, nuts and grass fed, raw dairy. Oysters, crab, and lobster have high levels of zinc, but they are so contaminated with pollutants that you may want to limit their use.

FAVORITE FOODS THAT WEAKEN CANCER

By now, I know that you have a whole new appreciation for the power of foods and how they influence our gene expression and ultimately our health. There are specific foods that seem to have more of an effect than others when it comes to preventing or healing Breast Cancer.

I recently watched a TED talk called *Foods That Starve Cancer*, presented by Dr. William LI.[441] I love his approach and reasoning since he recognizes that, "We are treating cancer too late in the game, when it is already established. Oftentimes, it's already spread." The tipping point or the development of cancer is often the formation of new blood vessels that feed tumors – angiogenesis. I have mentioned this many times throughout this book.

He reasoned, "What could we be adding to our diet that is naturally anti-angiogenic that would boost the body's defense system and beat back those blood vessels that are feeding the cancer?"

---

[439] https://www.levitamins.com/54692/ProductDetails?item=00915
[440] http://www.ncbi.nlm.nih.gov/pubmed/20155630
[441] http://www.ted.com/talks/william_li.html

I have discussed several nutrients that have been shown to have that ability but here is a partial list of some of the foods that have anti-angiogenic properties. You can see how many foods there are that can have this effect, IF we consume them regularly as part of our daily diet. This is a great reminder to view our food choices as a prescription for health - Essential #1: Let Food Be Your Medicine:

- Several fruits such as berries, citrus fruits, apples, cherries, and grapes.
- Red wine or resveratrol.
- Vegetables such as kale, Bok choy, artichokes, and parsley.
- Spices such as turmeric and nutmeg.
- Oils such as grape seed oil and olive oil.
- And lastly, 'la pièce de resistance,' dark chocolate ☺.

Here are more foods that you may find beneficial for you healing journey.

BAKING SODA

It may come as a surprise to many that plain old baking soda (sodium bicarbonate) would be part of a healing protocol. The beneficial use of baking soda can be explained with simple Chemistry 101.

Cancer cells have an acidic pH and thrive in an acidic environment.[442] Acidity in the tissues promote invasion and increases the spread of cancer cells.[443]

Normal, healthy blood pH is slightly on the alkaline side.

Introducing potent alkalizing liquids on a daily basis helps to alkalize the body fluids, making the environment unfavorable for cancer cell growth.[444] Bicarbonate inhibits the spread of Breast Cancer cells.[445]

---

[442] http://www.ncbi.nlm.nih.gov/pubmed/10362108
[443] http://www.ncbi.nlm.nih.gov/pubmed/23936808
[444] http://www.ncbi.nlm.nih.gov/pubmed/22704445
[445] http://www.ncbi.nlm.nih.gov/pubmed/19276390

Scientists have even seen more favorable results in the use of certain chemotherapy drugs when they increase the alkalinity of the drinking water with baking soda.[446]

Cancer research with sodium bicarbonate has suggested that it could play a major role in controlling the cellular pH in Breast Cancer tissues.[447] Because of the promising animal and lab results, Dr. Mark Pagel received a $2 million grant from the NIH to study the effectiveness of baking soda treatment for Breast Cancer.

However, the real Bicarbonate specialist is Dr. T. Simoncini.[448] Dr. Simoncini is an Italian oncologist who firmly believes that cancer is a fungus. Inject the tumor with a baking soda solution and the tumor shrivels up and dies. I consulted with a woman in Europe who visited Dr. Simoncini and had this procedure done to her large cancerous breast tumor. She applied the principles of The 7 Essentials along with Dr. Simoncini's protocol, and she is cancer free today!

In his book, *Cancer is a Fungus*[449], he details his theories and various protocols for different types of tumors.

If you want to increase your alkalinity, mix 1 teaspoon of baking soda in 8 ounces of water, several times per day, and drink up. Always do this at least 30 minutes before food or 2 hours after food, since this alkaline solution may neutralize the acids in your stomach.

There is a specific baking soda–maple syrup protocol named after Jim Kelmun. He apparently was a country doctor who experimented with natural medicines and found that baking soda was reversing many various types of cancer. Adding the maple syrup to the baking soda allows it to target the cancer cells first, since we know that cancer cells LOVE sugar. The Cancer Tutor has a simple explanation of the protocol.[450] Make sure you do this with the supervision of your health care practitioner.

---

[446] http://www.ncbi.nlm.nih.gov/pubmed/10362108
[447] http://www.ncbi.nlm.nih.gov/pubmed/22907202
[448] http://www.curenaturalicancro.com/
[449] http://www.cancerisafungus.com/
[450] http://www.cancertutor.com/what_to_do_today/

BUDWIG PROTOCOL

Dr. Johanna Budwig was a cancer researcher and biochemist who saved thousands of lives through her cancer programs. It has been said that her program has seen a 90% success rate over a 50 year period.

Dr. Budwig recommended that people changed their eating habits and consumed a mixture of cottage cheese and flax oil several times per day. Her disease cures are well documented and have withstood the test of opposition from mainstream medicine.

Because of her background in biochemistry, she realized that trans fats and hydrogenated vegetable oils from processed foods were 'dead' oils that clogged the cell membrane and changed the electrical charge in the cell. Without the proper charge, the cells were suffocating from lack of oxygen and proper nutrients.

Her formula of flax seed oil, a highly unsaturated fatty acid, combined with sulfur rich proteins actually made the flax oil water soluble, allowing it to be easily absorbed into the cell. This re-established the healthy charge to the cell so that it could 'breathe' again.

Here is the recipe from the Budwig Center in Spain:[451]

Budwig Diet Flaxseed Oil and Cottage Cheese (FOCC) or quark recipe:

Generally, each tablespoon of Flaxseed Oil (FO) is blended with 2 or more tablespoons of low-fat organic Cottage Cheese (CC) or quark.

NOTE: Whenever tablespoons are mentioned it is the standard United States tablespoon, which is the equivalent of the British 'dessert' spoon. 1 United States tablespoon = 15 ml and 1 British tablespoon is 18 ml - 16 tablespoons = cup and 4 tablespoons = 1/4 cup.

To make the Budwig Muesli:

- Blend 3 tablespoons (British dessert spoons) of flaxseed oil (FO) with 6 Tbsps. low-fat (less than 2%) Quark or Cottage Cheese (CC) with a hand-held immersion electric blender for up to a minute. If the mixture is too thick and/or the oil does not disappear you may need to add 2 or 3 tablespoons of milk (goat milk would be the best option). Do not add water or juices when blending FO with CC or quark. The mixture should be like rich whipped cream with no separated oil. Remember you must mix ONLY the FO and CC and nothing else at first. Always use organic food products when possible.
- Now once the FO and CC are well mixed, grind 2 Tbsps. of whole flaxseeds and add to the mixture. Please note that freshly ground flax seeds must be used within 20 minutes after being ground or they will become rancid. Therefore, do not grind up flaxseeds ahead of time and store.
- Next mix in by hand or with the blender 1 teaspoon of honey (raw non-pasteurized is recommended.) (Optional.)
- For variety you may add other ingredients such as sugar free apple sauce, cinnamon, vanilla, lemon juice, chopped almonds, hazelnuts, walnuts, cashews (no peanuts), pine kernels, or rosehip-marrow. For people who find the Budwig Muesli hard to take, these added foods will make the mixture more

[451] http://www.budwigcenter.com/the-budwig-diet.php

palatable. Some of our patients have even added a pinch of Celtic sea salt and others put in a pinch of cayenne pepper for a change.

- Add ground up Apricot kernels (no more than 6 kernels per day). Or you may decide to eat these apricot kernels on their own.

Skeptical at first, Dr. Dan C. Roehm, M.D., an oncologist and former cardiologist, tested and reviewed Dr. Budwig's protocol in the 1990s and concluded:

"This diet is far and away the most successful anti-cancer diet in the world. Cancer is easily curable. The treatment is dietary/lifestyle, the response is immediate; the cancer cell is weak and vulnerable; the precise biochemical breakdown point was identified by her in 1951 and is specifically correctable, in vitro (test tube) and as well as in vivo (real live body)...."

Personally, I could not get past the taste of the cottage cheese - flax oil combo and would have to say that is the biggest complaint that I hear from clients all over the world. Fortunately, I was introduced to a product that has organic, hormone-free powdered cottage cheese, combined with flax oil. It's called Celltra Max.[452] The products are dried at very low temperatures, which means they are still raw and have all the potent enzymes of the raw cottage cheese and flax oil. The capsules contain wheatgrass while the powdered packet forms do not.

I love them because they are handy and easy, especially if you travel and don't want to carry flax oil with you. Whether you are being proactive with prevention or if you are on a healing journey, consider adding the cottage cheese-flax oil mixture to your daily routine.

GARLIC

Garlic has long been known for its anti-bacterial, anti-fungal, and anti-viral properties.

---

452 http://breastcancerconquerorshop.com/product/procella/

The National Cancer Institute has a fact sheet about Garlic and Cancer Prevention that states, "Preliminary studies suggest that garlic consumption may reduce the risk of developing several types of cancer."[453]

Why aren't oncologists telling their patients to eat more garlic?

If the taste of garlic is an aversion, Kyolic carries an organically grown and aged garlic that converts the organo-sulfur compounds into effective compounds that are responsible for many health benefits.[454] The aging also removes the strong odor-causing agents so you don't have to worry about "garlic breath."

There are over 50 research papers on the effectiveness of garlic on cancer:

- Helps to detoxify carcinogens.[455]
- Garlic extract slows down the growth of Breast Cancer cells.[456]
- Inhibits tumor growth.[457]
- Breast Cancer cells are sensitive to the anti-cancer properties of garlic extract.[458]
- Reduces the side effects of chemotherapy.[459]

So how much is enough garlic per day? For general health, The World Health Organization suggests about 1 clove (2-5 grams) of fresh garlic or up to 1,000 mg of garlic extract per day. Obviously, with all the anti-cancer benefits, the more garlic the better.

---

[453] http://www.cancer.gov/cancertopics/factsheet/Prevention/garlic-and-cancer-prevention
[454] http://www.kyolic.com/
[455] http://www.ncbi.nlm.nih.gov/pubmed/23960721
[456] http://www.ncbi.nlm.nih.gov/pubmed/23050048
[457] http://www.ncbi.nlm.nih.gov/pubmed/23700562
[458] http://www.ncbi.nlm.nih.gov/pubmed/21428708
[459] http://www.ncbi.nlm.nih.gov/pubmed/21269259

GREEN POWDERS

Adding powdered greens to your smoothies or water will add more nutrient- dense power to your body. Since powdered greens are very concentrated, they are very alkalizing and filling. Only purchase raw, organic green powder. You will be wasting your money if you buy anything else. My favorite raw greens powder is from Garden of Life, but there are many excellent formulas to choose from.

MATCHA GREEN TEA

For many years I was aware that green tea had healing properties, but I never could get into the habit of drinking it regularly. And then I discovered Matcha Green Tea, the mother of all green teas.[460]

A study conducted at the University of Colorado reported that Matcha Green Tea has over 137 times more EGCG[461], a powerful anti-oxidant, than regular green tea.

Drinking 1 cup of Matcha is equivalent to drinking 10 cups of regular green tea.

Matcha has a higher ORAC score than blueberries and is loaded with trace minerals like selenium and zinc. The chlorophyll is a great detoxifier and is full of soluble and insoluble fibers that clean out the colon and the arteries. It has 5 times more L-Theanine, which is a great brain relaxer.

There are over 130 studies on the benefits of EGCG and Breast Cancer. Here are a few highlights:

- Suppression of Breast Cancer Stem Cells.[462]
- Targets tumor cells and inhibits the growth of new blood vessels that feed tumors (angiogenesis.)[463]

---

460 http://www.matchasource.com/?utm_source=Share+A+Sale&utm_medium=affiliate+ads&utm_campaign=Matcha+Source+Affiliates

461 http://www.ncbi.nlm.nih.gov/pubmed/14518774

462 http://www.ncbi.nlm.nih.gov/pubmed/22459208

463 http://www.ncbi.nlm.nih.gov/pubmed/23638734

- Reduces inflammatory factors in breast tissue.[464]
- Inhibits growth and spread of triple negative Breast Cancer.[465]
- Down-regulates estrogen on ER+ and PR+ Breast Cancer cells.[466]
- Induces cancer cell death in triple negative cancer.[467]

I enjoy 2 cups of Matcha every day. Sometimes, I even add a few teaspoons in my smoothies for that extra EGCG and anti-oxidant punch. You will love this web site[468] as it has great recipes and ideas on how to incorporate Matcha into your protocol. I also appreciate the fact that the founder and owner of the company, Alissa White[469], went to Japan to make sure the source was, in fact, organic and that the tea leaves were processed properly.

There have been some recent concerns about radiation contamination to the Matcha source. I have been assured by Alissa that the company in Japan tests the products, air, water and soil and have done so for decades. As of March, 2014, there were no detectable levels of radiation. Interestingly, acceptable levels by US standards are far higher than the Japanese.

WHEY PROTEIN

Whey protein is a high branched amino acid that rarely causes any dairy allergies. Casein, the protein in milk, is what causes most allergic reactions. Unfortunately, most whey proteins on the market have been heated at high temperatures and are processed from cows that have been injected with hormones and antibiotics.

---

[464] http://www.ncbi.nlm.nih.gov/pubmed/23880231
[465] http://www.ncbi.nlm.nih.gov/pubmed/23646788
[466] http://www.ncbi.nlm.nih.gov/pubmed/23322423
[467] http://www.ncbi.nlm.nih.gov/pubmed/23163783
[468] http://www.ncbi.nlm.nih.gov/pubmed/23163783
[469] http://www.matchasource.com/?utm_source=Share+A+Sale&utm_medium=affiliate+ads&utm_campaign=Matcha+Source+Affiliates

The cleanest and most potent RAW whey protein powder that I have found is from One World Whey.[470] Mike Adams from Natural News conducted a laboratory analysis of several whey proteins, including many plant protein powders, and found that One World Whey was by far the purest and cleanest whey on the planet.

I love whey protein because it maximizes glutathione[471] production by up to 64% and helps to normalize blood sugar[472] levels. Remember that glutathione is a primary anti-oxidant that detoxifies carcinogens and that is manufactured in your cells. It has been shown to inhibit the growth of cancer cells and stimulate your Natural Killer cells.[473]

Add whey protein to water, nut milks, or to your smoothies every day.

SUPPORTIVE THERAPIES

There are many various types of supportive therapies that have proven successful on a healing journey. These are a few that I believe are worth mentioning because of the results of patients who have incorporated these into their protocol:

IPT

IPT stands for Insulin Potentiation Therapy. IPT targets cancer cells with insulin and lower doses of chemotherapy. The lower doses often negate the destructive side effects or regular dosing of chemo.

We know that cancer cells have 17 times more insulin receptor sites compared to a regular cell. During the IPT treatment, a small amount of insulin is given to the patient to lower their blood sugar and then a low dose of chemotherapy is given by IV push. Giving the insulin 'fools' the cancer cells into thinking it is dinner time, when in fact, they are gobbling up the chemo.

---

470 http://www.sgn80.com/?a_aid=DrV
471 http://www.ncbi.nlm.nih.gov/pubmed/12537959
472 http://www.ncbi.nlm.nih.gov/pubmed/22995389
473 http://www.ncbi.nlm.nih.gov/pubmed/17430183

This is a therapy that should be done under medical supervision by a doctor that has been trained in this method.[474]

HYPERTHERMIA AND THE BIOMAT

Accumulating evidence indicates that physiological responses to Hyperthermia Therapy (HT) may impact the tumor environment through a variety of immunological responses.[475] In fact, in a Breast Cancer cell study, hyperthermia (105° degrees Fahrenheit or 42° degrees Celsius) was found to be slightly toxic to Breast Cancer cells and Breast Cancer Stem Cells, allowing improved target of a potential chemotherapeutic drug.[476]

Using a specific type of cell testing, scientists have found that hyperthermia disrupted the progression in Breast Cancer cells.[477] Combining nanoparticle-enhanced curcumin along with hyperthermia increased cancer cell destruction and death. The effectiveness of radiation and chemotherapy were enhanced using HT.

Clinical results achieved so far using hyperthermia should justify the use of this therapy as part of standard treatment for a tumor site. Significant improvements have been demonstrated using HT in a variety of cancers, including Breast Cancer.[478]

Remember that cancerous tissue has a low pH and thrives in an acidic environment. Treatments at temperatures between 40°-44° degrees Celsius (104° - 111° degrees Fahrenheit) prove toxic for cells in an environment of a low pH, which thus targets cancer cells and tumors.[479]

---

[474] http://www.ioicp.com/directory/cat/IPT/
[475] http://www.ncbi.nlm.nih.gov/pubmed/24490177
[476] http://www.ncbi.nlm.nih.gov/pubmed/24505341
[477] http://www.ncbi.nlm.nih.gov/pubmed/24511912
[478] http://www.ncbi.nlm.nih.gov/pubmed/12181239
[479] http://www.ncbi.nlm.nih.gov/pubmed/12181239

According to the National Cancer Institute, "Research has shown that high temperatures (up to 113° degrees Fahrenheit) can damage and kill cancer cells."[480]

Here are a few interesting facts from a book called, *The Fourth Medical Treatment of Medical Refugees*[481] by Nobuhiro Yoshimizu, M.D., Ph.D., former director of Yokohama General Hospital.

- Low body temperatures weaken the Immune System by 36% and reduces enzyme activity by 50%, which can eventually create an environment conducive to the growth of cancer cells. He found that 100% of his cancer patients had lower body temperatures.
- Thermotherapy kills cancer cells while improving the body's Immune System.
- Thermotherapy activates Heat Shock Proteins, (HSP) which activate Natural Killer cells and promote the synthesis of anti-cancer interferons.
- The production of endorphins as a result of the HSP production assists with pain control and stress reduction.
- Dr. Yoshimizu combines the Bio Mat Therapy with steam saunas and hot crystal infrared therapy to promote the synthesis of HSP.
- Dr. Yoshimizu uses the Biomat to weaken cancer cells and to reinforce the Immune System.
- The Biomat far infrared technology penetrates the body, up to 6 inches, affecting the lymph, organs, nerves, and vessels.
- Negative ions exist only in a clean environment. A lack of negative ions in the cells affects nutrition absorption and detoxification. As negative ions increase, the alkalinity of the body increases.

Download the FREE Ebook, *Thermotherapy in the New Century*, and learn more about the benefits and use of the BioMat.[482]

---

480 http://www.cancer.gov/cancertopics/factsheet/Therapy/hyperthermia
481 http://amzn.com/B0036USKX0

Although the BioMat provides far Infra-red therapy, it also has many other benefits:

- Increases circulation.
- Activates over 3000 essential enzymes.
- Lowers cortisol levels and stress in the body.
- Improves Immune function.
- Generates negative ions which open up the channels in the cell wall for improved nutrient and waste exchange.

I love my BioMat! Sleeping on it provides hours of negative, alkalizing ions being infused into my body.

TRANSDERMAL APPLICATION TO THE BREASTS

Your skin is the largest organ of the body. Anything you place on your skin is absorbed into the circulatory system and eventually ends up in your cells. Since the skin covering the breast tissue is very thin, application of specific substances may directly nourish the breast.

Do you take the time to love and nurture your breasts? It may sound silly, but our breasts are not just appendages on our chest or milk machines. They are an expression of our female-self and our nurturing qualities.

Whenever you bathe or shower, take a few extra minutes to massage the breast tissue in order to stimulate the lymphatic glands and tissues. Consider rotating the application of the following:

Magnesium chloride gel or oil

Iodine – you can 'paint' your breast with Lugol's Iodine. Be careful since the iodine will stain any clothing. Iodine has a clear anti-cancer effect on breast tumors.[483]

Cannibinoid Cream (Dixie Botanicals has a great product.[484])

---

[482] http://drv.biomat.com/

[483] http://www.ncbi.nlm.nih.gov/pubmed/17956159

Far Infra-Red Heat with the BioMat technology - hyperthermia kills cancer cells.

Exposure to Sunlight for 30 minutes per day.

Clay Packs – Clay poultices have a 'drawing effect' on toxins and heavy metals.

Oil of Frankincense - This extract has been shown to have anti-inflammatory and anti-neoplastic effects. Make sure you purchase a good quality oil since this can make all the difference in the effectiveness of the phyto-compounds. If you are on a healing journey, a concentrated form of frankincense is best. If you are being proactive with prevention, this ***Healthy Girls Breast Oil is lovely***.[485] It has frankincense as well as other oils that support breast health.

PUTTING IT ALL TOGETHER

At this point, you are probably on 'overload' with all this information and research. It was very important to me that you know that the principles of Natural Medicine are evidence-based. This can impart confidence in your natural preventive or healing protocol.

The big question is, "How do I apply this to my daily routine?" It does take a bit of organization and planning at first but once you have your game plan figured out, it simply becomes part of your routine. If you get frustrated, take a deep breath and be thankful for the knowledge that you have about Natural Medicines. Be thankful for your ability to purchase them and have them in your home. Be thankful that you have the strength to carry out a game plan. Be thankful for all the life-enhancing bio-chemical reactions that will occur as a result of applying The 7 Essentials.

When you focus on the power and the benefits of engaging in a healing routine, the motivation comes easily. When I was on my healing journey, I expressed gratitude daily, and multiple times

---

484 http://dixiebotanicals.com/products/salvation-balm/
485 http://breastcancerconquerorshop.com/product/healthy-girls-breast-oil/

during the day, that I had the opportunity to heal at home rather than having to lie in a hospital bed plugged into an IV drip.

Which brings me to this next thought: just because you are healing at home does not mean that you can continue with your hectic schedule as 'Super-mom'. To me, healing is a family affair. Inform the children that 'Mom' is healing her body, and she needs extra rest and a bit of relief from all of her regular activities. Herbal chemo is potent, and your body is using up lots of energy and resources to heal and detox the dead cancer cells.

Organize your juices and your supplements. Set your timer for your teas and tinctures. ***Schedule mindful meditations***. Commit to doing your coffee enemas every day. This is necessary for a successful outcome. If you feel overwhelmed one day, call your best friend and let her know that you need a day out at the movies or something. Relax and read a book that will enthrall you and inspire you. Or spend time outside, enjoying the sunshine and the fresh air.

Let's look at what a typical day may look like if you are on a healing journey. This is an example only and is not intended as a set protocol.

UPON AWAKENING:

Before brushing your teeth or drinking water, test your morning saliva pH and urinary pH.

Start your day with a glass of clean water with the juice of 1 lemon, powdered Vitamin C, and powdered magnesium. If you are taking enzymes every hour on the hour, this is a good time to start. Set your timer for hourly reminders.

The next liquid can be either Haelan or a mixture of Enduracell broccoli sprout powder in 4 ounces of water, or you might start with the Baking soda protocol. If you are doing the Baking soda, remember to wait at least 30 minutes before eating or drinking anything, including any enzymes or cancer-killing herbs.

Take your enzymes, Beta Glucans and your sublinguals such as DHEA and B 12.

Enjoy a short 20 -30 minute walk.

BREAKFAST:

Make your raw juice for the day. Enjoy 8 – 12 ounces of juice. Take your morning supplements.

Prepare the coffee for a coffee enema.

While doing your enema, you can listen to soothing relaxing music or a meditation CD.

Dry brush your body and shower.

After drying off, place magnesium oil on the soles of your feet and lower back and neck.

If you want a mid-morning brunch, now is a good time to have a raw whey protein shake or raw nuts.

Reading or meditation time is next in a far infrared sauna or while you lay on the BioMat. If those therapies are not available, try to sit near a window or outside in the sun.

Remember to be drinking plenty of clean, purified water. If you have added herbal tinctures to your journey, an easy way to make sure you get your proper dosage is by adding them to your drinking water and sip on them throughout the day.

If you are taking homeopathics, you can take them here, away from food. Wait at least 15 minutes before and after food and water when taking homeopathic remedies.

LUNCH TIME:

Lunch can include raw, green juice and a salad with a boiled egg. This is a good time to take the next dose of your supplements.

Remember to take your enzymes.

Whatever activities you plan for the afternoon, try to get some rest to nap or meditate again. A 20 minute power nap does your body good by recharging your batteries.

DINNER TIME

Dinner can include sautéed vegetables, raw soups, more salads, and a bit of protein. Time to take more of your supplements.

Remember to enjoy various teas such as Matcha, Chaga, or Essiac throughout the day. If you organize your time and supplements, it simply becomes part of your routine. As you see and feel improvement in your health, you will be more and more motivated to stick to your schedule.

Here is an overview of the 4 Categories. You can use this as a sample checklist to help you organize your healing journey. If you are not sure which products or protocols would be best for you, feel free to contact me with any questions.

Tumor Terminators:

- Blood Root and Enzymes
- Apricot Seeds and B 17
- Broccoli Sprouts powder
- Curcumin
- GcMAF
- Haelan 951 - Fermented soy
- Hemp oil and CBD
- Poly MVA
- Salicinium (also known as Orasal)
- Spirulina

Body Builders:

- Beta Glucans
- Chaga
- Essiac Tea
- Herbal and homeopathic support
- IP 6
- Probiotics

Nourishing Nutrients:

- DIM and I3C
- Glutathione
- Flax Seeds and Flax oil
- Iodine
- Magnesium
- Melatonin
- Omega 3 Fatty Acids
- Selenium
- Vitamin C
- Vitamin D
- Zinc

Favorite Foods:

- Baking Soda
- Budwig Protocol
- Garlic
- Greens powder
- Matcha Green Tea
- Whey Protein

Supportive Therapies:

- IPT
- Hyperthermia with the BioMat or infrared sauna
- Transdermal applications to the breasts

POINTS TO PONDER

This has been a very full chapter with a lot of information. You may want to review this chapter several times to be clear about what feels right for you.

- The National Library of Medicine provides an abundance of evidence-based research about natural medicines.
- The phytochemicals in Blood Root have many anti-cancer properties.
- Enzyme therapy has anti-tumor and anti-metastatic effects.
- Apricot seeds contain a sugar-complex-cyanide that is toxic to cancer cells but harmless to healthy cells. Another example of selective toxicity.
- Broccoli sprouts contain sulforaphane which kills Breast Cancer cells and enhances your Natural Killer Cell activity.
- There are over 200 studies on the benefits of Curcumin and Breast Cancer.
- Japanese research about GcMAF demonstrates that it activates the Mack Truck Macrophages to gobble up cancer cells.
- Fermented soy converts cancer stem cells to normal healthy stem cells.
- CBD oil is the first non-toxic agent that significantly decreases the expression of metastatic Breast Cancer.
- Salicinium, also known as Orasal, is a sugar based molecule that interrupts the fermentation process of cancer cells.
- Poly MVA is a unique formulation that interferes with the cancer cells' metabolism.
- Three to four teaspoons of Spirulina has been shown to have anti-cancer effects.
- It is important to weaken the cancer but at the same time you must support and boost your Immune System.
- Beta Glucans found in medicinal mushrooms stimulate and activate macrophages that gobble up cancer cells.

- Essiac tea has been shown to have anti-cancer properties.
- Herbal tincture and homeopathy are a powerful adjunct to any preventive and healing protocol.
- IP6 is another natural medicine that directly affects the metabolism of cancer cells and has inhibited the growth of Breast Cancer cells by 50%.
- Probiotics stimulate anti-tumor immunity in Breast Cancer models.
- Compounds found in cruciferous vegetables called DIM I3C help convert and metabolize aggressive estrogens into benign estrogens.
- Increasing glutathione production with curcumin, broccoli sprouts, and raw whey boosts the detoxification pathways.
- Adding 5 teaspoons of ground flax seeds reduced tumor markers by 30% to 71%.
- Iodine appears to be a requisite of healthy breast tissue.
- Magnesium deficiency seems to be carcinogenic, while high magnesium levels inhibit carcinogenesis.
- Melatonin triggers cancer cell death.
- Omega 3 fatty acids from walnuts, clean fish, and flax decrease the growth rate of Breast Cancer cells.
- Vitamin D decreased overall cancer risk by as much as 77%.
- Vitamin C has been shown to slow the growth and spread of several types of cancer.
- Low levels of Selenium may be associated with the development of Breast Cancer.
- There are specific foods that block the formation of blood vessels that feed tumors.
- Baking Soda alkalizes the body. Cancer cells are acidic and don't like alkalinity.
- The Budwig protocol has a 90% success rate over a 50 year period.

- Garlic has many anti-cancer properties.
- 1 cup of Matcha green tea is equivalent to 10 cups of regular green tea.
- Hyperthermia boosts the Immune System and weakens cancer cells.
- Love those girls (your breasts) by massaging various applications of oils and minerals.

YOUR HEALING JOURNEY ACTION STEPS

- ➢ Become familiar with the many evidence-based supplements and foods that boost your Immune System and weaken the cancer cells.
- ➢ Re-read this chapter several times and decide what protocols work best for you.
- ➢ Take a moment to organize your time for your healing journey.
- ➢ Start eating apricot kernels every day.
- ➢ Add Broccoli Sprouts and Spirulina to your water or juice every day.
- ➢ Enjoy various teas throughout the day.
- ➢ Grind 5 teaspoons of flax seeds and enjoy them on salads or in your smoothies.
- ➢ Apply magnesium oil to the soles of your feet, lower back, and neck.
- ➢ Try to get at least 1 hour of sunshine on your body and eyeballs every day.
- ➢ Measure your saliva and urine pH first thing in the morning. Your saliva should be more alkaline than your urine.
- ➢ Add raw, organic, whey protein to your juice or smoothies to help boost your glutathione production.
- ➢ Sit in a far infrared sauna for 30 to 45 minutes several times per week.

- Relax on a BioMat for at least 1 hour per day. Sleep on it all night if you own one.
- Meditate and visualize your natural medicines boosting your Immune System and weakening the cancer cells, creating a vibrant, healthier you.

CHAPTER 8

ESSENTIAL #7 – ADOPT VERY EARLY DETECTION

"Let's face it. In America today we don't have a health care system, we have a sick care system."

~

Tom Harkins, U.S. Senator

Early detection is by far the best plan to circumvent Breast Cancer. I love working with women who are being proactive with prevention. They are inquisitive and are searching for better ways to improve their overall health, which ultimately improves their breast health.

If you rely only on the advice of a traditional mainstream medical doctor, chances are that your 'bill of health' will be short-lived. We have all heard the stories of someone getting a 'complete checkup' with a clean bill of health and the next day they drop dead of a heart attack. According to the WHO, "Cancer cases are expected to surge 57% worldwide in the next 20 years."[486]

---

486 http://www.cnn.com/2014/02/04/health/who-world-cancer-report/index.html?hpt=hp_t2

If you have the "This will never happen to me" attitude, think again. ***As of 2014, 1 out of 3 women and 1 out 2 men are destined to develop some form of cancer.*** We live in a toxic and stressed out world with nutrient deficient food. Our Immune Systems are weakened by the onslaught of chemicals and stress hormones that we release because of our hectic lifestyles. We swim in a soup of Electro-pollution that causes DNA damage.

Unless you are proactive and become conscious of your long-term health, you may face the diagnosis of cancer. In this chapter, I will focus on specific blood and urine tests that may give you years of warning, way before you find a lump or a bump.

The pink frenzy with Breast Cancer Awareness Month, has done absolutely nothing to raise awareness about **true prevention** of Breast Cancer.

Instead of educating women about diet, toxic exposures, emotional healing, and dental toxicities, it promotes mammography screening and drug-related approaches. If you follow the basic principles outlined in The 7 Essentials, you may never have to fear cancer again.

Let's start with the biggest multi-billion dollar 'screening' tool, mammography. In this section, I am presenting you with the facts. I am not suggesting that you never have a mammogram. That is your choice. And to be fair, I have heard from women who never knew they had Breast Cancer until they had a mammogram. Ultimately, you weigh the risks with the benefits and decide what is best for you.

THE BIG SQUEEZE AND THE MAMMOGRAM MYTH

Let's begin with the largest and most meticulous study of mammography ever done.[487] This was a 25 year study, published in the *British Medical Journal*, February 2014, of Canadian women from the ages of 40 to 59.

---

[487] http://www.nytimes.com/2014/02/12/health/study-adds-new-doubts-about-value-of-mammograms.html?_r=0

The conclusion of the study said:[488]

"Annual mammography in women aged 40-59 does NOT REDUCE MORTALITY FROM BREAST CANCER beyond that of physical examination..."

According to Cornell University's Program on Breast Cancer and Environmental Risk Factors, "Female breast tissue is highly susceptible to radiation effects."[489] The American Cancer Society states, "...Mammograms do not work as well in women with dense breasts, since dense breasts can hide a tumor."[490]

"By the time Breast Cancer is detected on a mammogram, a woman will have already had the disease for an average of 6 to 8 years."

(American Cancer Society, 2001.)

In a press release through World Wire.com, Dr. Samuel Epstein, a renowned advocate for cancer prevention and Dr. Rosalie Bertell, founding member of the European Committee on Radiation Risk, stated:[491]

"Routine mammography delivers an unrecognized high dose of radiation. If a woman follows the current guidelines for premenopausal screening, over a 10 year period she would receive a total dosage of about 5 rads. This approximates the level of exposure to radiation of a Japanese woman one mile from the epicenter of atom bombs dropped on Hiroshima or Nagasaki."

In a study published in the *British Journal of Radiology* researchers found compelling evidence that low energy X-rays used in mammograms are "approximately 4 times, but possibly as much as 6 times more effective in *causing mutational damage* than higher

---

488 http://www.ncbi.nlm.nih.gov/pubmed/24519768

489 http://envirocancer.cornell.edu/factsheet/physical/fs52.radiation.cfm

490 http://www.cancer.org/cancer/breastcancer/moreinformation/breastcancerearlydetection/breast-cancer-early-detection-acs-recs-mammograms

491 http://www.world-wire.com/news/0911240002.html

energy X-rays."[492] In other words, the low energy radiation is causing DNA damage that could result in an increased risk of developing Breast Cancer.

In a Norwegian study that followed 2 various groups of women for 5 years, researchers reported that women who had mammograms every 2 years had 22% more Breast Cancers compared to the group who just had 1 screening in 6 years.[493] Could the radiation be responsible for the increase in Breast Cancer?

False positives are also of great concern. The cumulative risk of false-positives increases to as high as 100% over a decade's screening for women with multiple high-risk factors such as strong family history and prolonged use of the contraceptive pill.[494] Think of the psychological and physical trauma of being falsely diagnosed resulting in multiple biopsies and more mammograms.

Participants in a study about the psychological consequences of 'false-positive' mammograms shared psycho-social outcomes at various monthly intervals.[495] ***The conclusion of the study was, "False-positive findings on screening mammography causes long-term psycho-social harm."*** Three years after a 'false-positive' diagnosis, the psycho-social behaviors that were affected were: feelings of dejection, anxiety, attractiveness, worries of Breast Cancer, as well as negative impact on sleep, behavior, and sexuality.

Over-diagnosing often leads to over-treatment, which is another major risk of regular mammograms. A prime example is in the case of DCIS, a 0 grade and 'non-cancer'. Although some 80% of untreated DCIS never become invasive, it is often aggressively treated with a lumpectomy, mastectomies, radiation, and chemotherapy. Early detection of DCIS with mammograms does NOT reduce mortality as confirmed by a 13 year Canadian study.[496]

---

[492] http://www.ncbi.nlm.nih.gov/pubmed/?term=16498030

[493] http://www.nytimes.com/2008/11/25/health/25breast.html?ref=health&pagewanted=all&_r=0

[494] http://jnci.oxfordjournals.org/content/92/20/1657.long

[495] http://www.annfammed.org/content/11/2/106.long

[496] http://www.ncbi.nlm.nih.gov/pubmed/10995804

The researchers at Green Med Info.com[497], have spent considerable time indexing research form the National Library of Medicine about the adverse effects of radiation from mammograms. It is an excellent source of evidence-based Natural Medicine. I encourage you to read the research instead of relying on mainstream medicine and flashy news reporting.

Not only is their increased risk from the radiation exposure, but there is an increased cancer risk from the often painful compression[498] of the mammography machine. The compression can lead to rupturing of small tumors and blood vessels, spreading malignant cancer cells throughout the body.

Personal and regular breast exams are a safe and effective alternative[499] to mammograms. ***In 1985, the American Cancer Society admitted that "at least 90% of women who discover breast carcinoma discover the tumor themselves."*** In a pooled analysis of several studies[500], women who regularly performed Breast Self-Exams (BSE) detected the breast tumors much earlier and with fewer lymph node involvement.

In spite of all the facts, the American Cancer Society and the billion dollar mammogram industry continue to lure women of all ages into hospitals and mammogram centers. It is unconscionable that the cancer industry continues to capture unsuspecting and trusting women into the grips of radiation and painful compression.

Dr. Epstein's web site, Cancer Prevention Coalition[501], exposes the cancer industry's cash cows such as the American Cancer Society and its close ties with the mammography industry and the profitable, cancer drugs manufacturer, Big Pharma.

---

497 http://www.greenmedinfo.com/affiliate/2929/node/53664

498 http://onlinelibrary.wiley.com/doi/10.1002/14651858.CD002942.pub2/full

499 http://www.preventcancer.com/patients/mammography/ijhs_mammography.htm

500 http://www.ncbi.nlm.nih.gov/pubmed/?term=J.+Natl.+Cancer+Inst.+85(7)%3A+525-526%2C+1993

501 http://www.preventcancer.com/losing/acs/wealthiest_links.htm

THERMOGRAPHIC IMAGING

Thermography, also known as Digital Infrared Thermographic Imaging (DITI), offers the opportunity of very early detection of breast disease over and above self-breast exams and mammography alone. Is it 100% accurate all of the time? No. But neither are mammograms and self- breast exams.

Thermography is a non-invasive test of physiology that can alert your doctor to changes that could indicate early stages of breast disease. When used in conjunction with other procedures, the best possible evaluation of breast health is made.[502]

Here is an over simplification of how DITI works:

- Our body emits heat that is picked up and recorded with the DITI camera.
- When there is inflammation, there is more heat that is generated. (Think of a swollen ankle or knee after a sports injury)
- More heat is registered by the camera and translated into an image through specialized, computer software.
- Increased inflammation in the breast can be a result of angiogenesis, or the formation of new blood vessels that are feeding a tumor. With increasing evidence that inflammation often enhances tumor growth, DITI may have considerable beneficial value[503] in the prognosis due to early detection.
- These abnormal heat patterns[504] are among the earliest signs of a developing cancer, according to Dr. William Hobbins, M.D., a board certified thermologist and Fellow of the American Board of Surgeons. He has been performing DITI for over 35 years.

---

502 http://thermologyonline.org/Research/Breast/Case%20Study.pdf

503 http://thermologyonline.org/Research/Scientific/Angiogenesis%20animal%20tumours.pdf

504 http://thermologyonline.org/Research/Breast/beating-breast-cancer.pdf

In a study conducted at the University of Louis Pasteur[505] in France, research scientists concluded that "Thermography is useful not only as a predictor of risk factor for cancer but also to assess the more rapidly growing neoplasms."

Angiogenesis[506] is present in more than 90% of non-palpable tumors and 100% of palpable lesions, according to Dr. P. Gamagami, MD, a radiologist at the Breast Center in Van Nuys, CA. He found that increased vascularity from enlarged arteries as vascular markers for Breast Cancers as small as 5 mm (0.2 inches). His group has found that tumor angiogenesis causes "hot spots in the affected breast, even in the absence of recognized signs of developing cancer."

This is very encouraging information for Breast Cancer prevention and treatment. Imagine being able to proactively lower the inflammatory levels with lifestyle changes and epigenetic nutrition in order to nip the cancer in the bud. Think of the impact this could have on Breast Cancer mortality rates, since 80% of Breast Cancers that are discovered are already a palpable mass.

Thermography's key asset[507] is that it seems to spot active pre-cancerous breast signs some 6 – 8 years before any palpable mass appears.

Other than very early detection, DITI offers many other benefits. There is NO radiation, NO compression, NO pain, and NO touching.

According to guidelines set by the FDA, thermography is not a replacement for screening mammography and should not be used by itself to diagnose Breast Cancer. The American College of Clinical Thermography[508] clarifies the role of DITI by stating, "Thermography is not an alternative to mammography. Thermal imaging is a test of function and physiology and not structure and anatomy.

---

505 http://thermologyonline.org/Research/Breast/breast%20thermography%20and%20cancer%20risk%20prediction.pdf

506 http://thermologyonline.org/Research/Breast/Angiogenisis.pdf

507 http://thermologyonline.org/Research/Breast/thermography%20secret%20weapon.pdf

508 http://thermologyonline.org/index.html

Thermography is cleared as an adjunctive diagnostic test.... and can evaluate the physiological status of the body."

To learn more about the benefits of Thermography and to find ACCT approved Thermography Clinics, visit the American College of Clinical Thermography.[509]

VERY SENSITIVE BLOOD TESTS

The traditional cancer marker blood tests that are run for Breast Cancer are CA 15-3, CA 27.29, and CEA, a marker for the presence of Lung, Colon, and Liver Cancer, to see if the Breast Cancer has spread. Unfortunately these markers are not always reliable, as I have often seen women with active Breast Cancer with 'normal' cancer markers. These tests measure less well-defined cancer proteins or antigens and tend to be inconsistent, being elevated only in the late stage of the disease.

If the highly sensitive blood tests were part of the normal screening process, I believe that so many lives would be saved. Would it not be advantageous to the patient to discover cancer production on a cellular level instead of discovering it as a tumor in an advanced stage? Many countries are making use of this sensitive technology and are moving forward with scientific evidence that they are beneficial and can prevent suffering and save lives.

Remember that none of these tests are 'diagnostic' in themselves. The only way cancer can be truly diagnosed is with a biopsy and tissue sample of the area in question.

Some of these tests can be found grouped together in the Cancer Profiles[510] performed by American Metabolic Testing Laboratories. You can have these kits delivered to your home and have the blood drawn through your doctor's lab or any other public lab that offers that service.

---

509 http://thermologyonline.org/index.html

510 http://breastcancerconquerorshop.com/?s=TK1&post_type=product

The following tests are listed alphabetically.

AMAS

This test, performed by Oncolabs[511] in Boston, MA, measures a well-defined antibody whose serum levels rise early in the course of the disease. The AMAS test measures serum levels of AMA, an antibody found to be elevated in most patients with a wide range of active, non-terminal malignancies.

The limitation of this test is that a low AMA level can occur in non-cancer, in advanced and terminal cancer, and in successfully treated cancer.

CTC – CIRCULATING TUMOR CELLS

Circulating Tumor Cells (CTCs) in the blood are cells that have broken off from the main tumor and their presence is an indication that the cancer is spreading.

DHEA-S

This is a hormone produced by the adrenal glands that plays a vital role in hormonal balance and youthful vitality. According to Dr. Schandl of American Metabolic Laboratories[512], DHEA-S is an anti-stress, pro-immunity, and longevity hormone. Studies have shown that low levels of DHEA-S are associated with inflammatory disorders, cardiovascular disease, and cancer. ***Most cancer patients and those that are developing cancer have low serum DHEA-S levels.***

GREECE TEST

This test had its origin in Greece by Dr. I. Papasotiriou[513], medical director of RGCG –Ltd. (Research Genetic Cancer Center.) This blood test uses state of the art technology to determine the genes that are responsible for the growth and survival of the tumor. It tests the

---

511 http://www.oncolabinc.com/index.php
512 http://americanmetaboliclaboratories.net/
513 http://www.atmctx.com/cancer-test/

chemo-sensitivity of Circulating Tumor Cells and Cancer Stem Cells to see which chemotherapies are most effective in killing off these cells. It also checks over 50 natural medicines and nutrients that can kill cancer cells and stimulate the Immune System. It will even determine if the cancer is sensitive to radiotherapy and hyperthermia.

I find it to be a very comprehensive test that gives much insight into what may work more effectively in healing the cancer. The downside of the test is the cost.

HCG

More frequently known as the 'pregnancy hormone', Human Chorionic Gonadotropin, (HCG), is also a 'malignancy hormone'. HCG has been described in many cancer types and is involved in the formation, spread, and immune escape of Breast Cancer.[514] The analysis performed by American Metabolic Laboratories[515] is an extremely sensitive test that measure 2 types of HCG in the blood and 1 in the urine.

A word of warning: There is a urine test that is performed outside the United States that measures urinary HCG. However, this test is a very gross test since it is NOT specific for HCG only but will also pick up other strands of hormones such as TSH, (Thyroid), LH, and FSH. (Hormones found in a pre-menopausal woman).

It's your life. Don't take chances.

HOMOCYSTEINE

Although not related to cancer directly, high Homocysteine[516] may play an important role in Breast Cancer[517] development. Elevated

---

514 http://www.ncbi.nlm.nih.gov/pubmed/20654692
515 http://breastcancerconquerorshop.com/product-category/early-cancer-detection/
516 http://www.ncbi.nlm.nih.gov/pubmed/24023349
517 http://www.ncbi.nlm.nih.gov/pubmed/24166605

Homocysteine levels are associated with Breast Cancer progression.[518]

A few years ago, I discovered I had 'off the charts' high Homocysteine levels in spite of being an avid runner, exerciser, and excellent eater. I was shocked but grateful since that discovery opened up a whole new world and understanding of Breast Cancer. It was through that process that I discovered methylation and MTHFR gene mutation.

Homocysteine is an amino acid produced by the body as a by-product of protein breakdown. High levels are an indication that there is poor methylation or metabolic breakdown as a result of defective MTHFR genes, poor diet, and gastro-intestinal issues. High levels are associated with increased risk of stroke and cardiovascular disease but are also an indication that there may be a methylation issue, leading to improper estrogen metabolism.

HIGHLY SENSITIVE C REACTIVE PROTEIN

Although used specifically for cardiovascular disease, this test is a great indication of chronic inflammation in the body.[519] Studies have suggested a relationship between inflammation and post-menopausal Breast Cancer[520] risk, especially in women with excess adipose tissue.

NATURAL KILLER CELL ACTIVITY TEST

Natural Killer Cells are lymphocytes that respond to cells infected with viruses and to the formation of tumors. They can also produce chemicals that directly kill cancer cells. The stronger your NK cells, the stronger your Immune System.

ONCOBLOT

This is a highly sensitive test that identifies the presence of cancer through the detection of a growth related protein that is generated

---

518 http://www.ncbi.nlm.nih.gov/pubmed/23934182
519 https://circ.ahajournals.org/content/103/13/1813.full
520 http://www.ncbi.nlm.nih.gov/pubmed/24504436

solely by malignant cells.[521] It accurately determines the presence of 2 million cancer cells versus 4.5 trillion cells in an established tumor. It can reveal the tissue origin in over 26 different types of cancer. This can be a great test to find out if you are making cancer cells. The downside is that it is a little pricey.

PHI

This enzyme, secreted by cancer cells, regulates anaerobic metabolism, which is metabolism with sugar and not oxygen. It is also described as the Autocrine Motility Factor and plays a major factor as a malignancy promoter.[522] This is included in the Cancer Profile[523] by American Metabolic Laboratories.

THYROID PANEL

Detecting low thyroid activity is very important for prevention and healing of Breast Cancer.[524] A high TSH (Thyroid Stimulation Hormone) may indicate that the thyroid is sluggish and not responding to stimulation. A helpful thyroid panel would include TSH, T4, T3, and Free T4.

TK1 ENZYME

TK1 is an enzyme that is released during cell division and DNA repair. In healthy cells, TK1 is absorbed by the cell and is NOT released in the blood stream. This test is backed by over 30 years of research and hundreds of peer-reviewed research papers documenting a correlation between TK1 production and a variety of cancers, including Breast Cancer.[525] Elevated TK1 was found to be significantly elevated in Breast Cancer patients compared to healthy women.[526]

---

521 http://www.oncoblotlabs.com/
522 http://www.ncbi.nlm.nih.gov/pubmed/3085086
523 http://breastcancerconquerorshop.com/product-category/early-cancer-detection/
524 http://breastcancerconqueror.com/the-thyroid-breast-cancer-connection/
525 http://www.ncbi.nlm.nih.gov/pubmed/22778736
526 http://www.ncbi.nlm.nih.gov/pubmed/21178264

VITAMIN D

Higher serum levels of Vitamin D3 are associated with lower cancer risks and improved survival rates. You can ask your doctor to include this test in your regular blood work or you can order a simple spot test that you can do in the privacy of your home.[527]

GENOMIC TESTING

Genomic Testing or DNA testing[528] evaluates genetic variants and gives you a glimpse into the potential of a healthy or diseased future. The old school of thought was you inherited 'bad' genes from your parents and you inevitably acquired the disease. The new paradigm shift, thanks to the advances in Epigenetics, tells us that our genes may predispose us to a particular disease, but we have the power to change that expression with specific nutrients and lifestyle changes.

DNA testing will allow you to create preventative strategies and point to specific nutrients that would give you optimal support. It will reveal your body's anti-oxidant defense as being weak or strong. It can evaluate your inflammatory responses and how well your body can detoxify environmental toxins. It will help you understand your hormonal metabolic pathways and how your body responds to stress.

DNA testing is definitely the preventive medicine of the future.

SALIVA TESTS

Saliva testing measures the hormones that are bio-available versus the hormones in the blood that are attached to a protein. These protein-bound hormones comprise 95% of the hormones in the blood, yet they are bio-unavailable. They don't fit in the 'key-hole' of the receptor site on the cell.

Conversely, hormones that can be filtered through the salivary glands are not bound to a large protein and have been shown to be more bio-

---

527 http://breastcancerconquerorshop.com/product/vitamin-d-blood-drop-test/
528 http://smartdna.com.au/

available and thus represent a more accurate picture of hormone levels.

Saliva can reveal the balance of many intricate systems of your body, including your hormones, adrenal function, and neurotransmitters. These hormones are functionally interrelated, meaning that one set of hormones affects the other. If one is out of balance, it will cascade into creating imbalance with the others. Although the saliva tests are not 'diagnostic' as far as a cancer diagnosis, they give you much insight as to the stress that may have led to the development of Breast Cancer. Saliva testing may be useful if you are experiencing some of the following symptoms:

- Depression and anxiety
- Insomnia and fatigue
- Chronic illness and immune deficiencies
- PMS, menopause and andropause (yes, men go through menopause, too)
- Weight gain and thyroid issues

The most important tests to consider are the Comprehensive Saliva PLUS Panel[529] or the Neuro-Hormone PLUS Panel. If you are having issues with sleep, depression, foggy brain, and anxiety, the Neuro-Hormone Complete Sleep Panel PLUS[530] is the panel to consider.

URINE TESTS

- Essential Estrogen Urinalysis[531] is designed to assess the risk of estrogen-related diseases. This 24 hour home based urine test measures various estrogens and estrogen metabolites. It will indicate whether or not you are breaking down and metabolizing estrogen properly. If you are not methylating

---

529 http://breastcancerconquerorshop.com/product/comprehensive-saliva-plus-panel/

530 http://breastcancerconquerorshop.com/product/neuro-hormone-complete-panel/

531 http://breastcancerconquerorshop.com/product/estrogens-urinalysis-essential/

estrogen properly, the accumulation of the more aggressive estrogen may result in an increased risk of Breast Cancer.

- Urine Iodine testing[532] is a simple test that you can do in the privacy of your home. As discussed in Chapter 7, iodine is an anti-proliferative agent and contributes to the health of normal breast tissue. Low iodine levels and weak thyroids have been connected to an increase in Breast Cancer. Iodine testing is fundamental to prevention and healing of Breast Cancer.

This simple home test consists of collecting your urine for 24 hours after ingesting Iodoral tablets. Too little iodine in the urine means that your body is absorbing the iodine which may indicate a possible deficiency.

Of course there are many more valid tests that can be implemented in your preventative or healing regime. These are the tests that I have found beneficial in revealing key imbalances that may be contributing to ill health. As advances are made in integrated oncology practices, hopefully tests like these will be regularly recommended and prescribed.

POINTS TO PONDER

- According to a 2014 report by the World Health Organization, cancer cases are expected to surge over 57% worldwide.
- 1 out of 3 women and 1 out of 2 men are destined to develop some form of cancer in their lifetime.
- True prevention involves applying all the principles in The 7 Essentials.
- Mammograms do NOT reduce Breast Cancer mortality rates.
- Routine mammography, over a 10 year period, delivers the amount of exposure of radiation equivalent to what a Japanese woman was exposed to 1 mile from the epicenter of the atom bomb in Hiroshima.

---

532 http://breastcancerconquerorshop.com/product/urine-iodine-testing/

- Physical and psychological damages from 'false positives' mammograms have caused irreparable damage to millions of women.
- Compression from a mammogram can potentially rupture small tumors and cause malignant cells to spread throughout the body.
- Abnormal heat patterns are among the earliest signs of developing cancer.
- Thermography is a test of physiology and can be a key asset in spotting changes 6 -8 years before any palpable mass appears.
- There are several very sensitive blood tests that can detect the development of cancer at an early stage, before a tumor mass appears.
- Chronic inflammation may increase post-menopausal Breast Cancer risk.
- Low thyroid function has been associated with increased Breast Cancer risk.
- The TK1 enzyme test has been successfully used for over 30 years in 30 countries. Elevated TK1 enzymes levels were found to be significantly higher in Breast Cancer patients.
- Genomic or DNA testing can help you target specific strategies to support your health and improve the healing ability of your body.
- Saliva tests measure the hormones that are 'bio-available'.

YOUR HEALING JOURNEY ACTION STEPS

- Make a conscious decision to be proactive with prevention by following The 7 Essentials.
- Review the referenced links about mammography and make an informed decision about future screenings.
- Read up on Thermography on the ACCT web site. Find a certified Thermographer in your area and ask questions.
- Decide which preventive blood tests would work best for you and your budget.
- Next time you have regular blood work done through your medical doctor, ask about adding Homocysteine and the highly sensitive C reactive Protein test.
- Make sure your Vitamin D3 levels are in the upper range, near 80 ng/ml.
- Learn more about Genomic testing and add it to your bucket list.
- If you are being proactive with prevention, many of the suggested tests may provide information so that you can specifically target your health challenges.
- If you are on a healing journey, many of the suggested tests can give you a base line to help you measure the progress you are making.

EPILOGUE

THE END IS SIMPLY THE BEGINNING

"Just when the caterpillar thought the world was over... it became a butterfly."

~

Proverb

There are no accidents in the flow of life. We are energetic beings that are living in a Universe that vibrates and is moving at the speed of light. Coming into contact with this book was an indication that you were ready to receive and learn new principles of health.

If you have in fact read through all the material and have taken the time to read some of the cited references, you now have a greater understanding of the irrefutable Laws of Nature. Disease can only manifest itself when your body is out of balance and has tipped the scale to ill health.

Remember you do not get sick because you have cancer. You were already sick and THEN you developed cancer.

The Laws of Nature are very forgiving and very loving. All we have to do to restore health in the body is to be in sync with the natural laws and treat our bodies and minds with respect.

When I chose the purple butterfly for my personal and professional logo, (or should I say when the butterfly chose me ☺), it was such a peaceful moment. I was so grateful for everything that my healing journey had taught me. I learned to live with joy and a state of happiness that was constant. I became kind to myself. I forgave myself. I let go of the past and released the 'stories' that no longer served me.

I discovered balance and a renewed sense of purpose. I took the time to meditate and pray. I trained my brain and my mind to visualize and feel my ideal life of health, wealth, and laughter.

For years, I was chomping at the bit to begin writing this book. There were many times when I thought I was ready but things would not come together for me. I obviously had more to learn and to experience before I could share my message in a bigger way. Then, about a year ago, the pieces of the puzzle came together for me to begin and finally complete this information.

This book is a 'work of heart'. I know that I may not be the most expressive and eloquent writer. What I have endeavored to create, however, is a book that will fill you with hope. Knowledge is power, and my prayer for you is that one thought or one Essential from this book shifts your life for the better. If that happens, then my mission has been accomplished.

Whether you want to prevent Breast Cancer or whether you are on a healing journey with Breast Cancer, the underlying message is the same. You can learn to heal your body on all levels. Nourish your body, calm your mind, and nurture your soul and chances are you will heal and recover.

Remember that healing is a journey with no ultimate destination. It may be baby steps at first but if you push forward with faith and courage, you will emerge as a beautifully transformed 'new you'. Just as the cocoon may feel dark and cramped and afraid of what is next, the cocoon trusts the process and the Laws of Nature. With that trust and patience, it emerges as a totally transformed and elegant new being.

You, too, can trust the Laws of Nature by applying The 7 Essentials. In doing so, I pray that your life is filled with vibrant health and a renewed sense of joyful living.

With much love and gratitude,

Dr. V.

Sources & References

CHAPTER 1

http://appreciativeinquiry.case.edu/practice/organizationDetail.cfm?coid=852&sector=32 19
http://archsurg.jamanetwork.com/article.aspx?articleid=396893 37
http://articles.mercola.com/sites/articles/archive/2012/02/18/dangers-of-root-canaled-teeth.aspx 31
http://articles.mercola.com/sites/articles/archive/2012/08/25/heavy-metal-electromagnetic-fields.aspx#_edn2 31
http://astore.amazon.com/breacancconq-20?node=2&page=3 25
http://bioinitiative.org/freeaccess/editors/what.htm 25
http://bioinitiative.org/freeaccess/index.htm 25
http://breastcancerconqueror.com/stop-breast-cancer-before-it-starts/ 38
http://breastcancerconqueror.com/store/products/category/hormone-testing/ 33
http://breastcancerconqueror.com/treatments-for-dcis-cause-cancer/ 34
http://breastcancerconquerorshop.com/product/estrogens-urinalysis-essential/ 118, 238
http://cancerres.aacrjournals.org/content/65/19/8583.full 32
http://dceg.cancer.gov/about/organization/programs-ebp/reb 34
http://ehtrust.org/books-publications/newsletters/ 26
http://en.wikipedia.org/wiki/History_of_cancer_chemotherapy 38
http://en.wikipedia.org/wiki/Oxidative_stress 28
http://en.wikipedia.org/wiki/Tamoxifen 39

http://www.miessence.com/miessenceStory/ingredientsWeShun?lang=en&here=miessenceStory/ingredientsWeShun 24
http://www.nature.com/bjc/index.html 36
http://www.ncbi.nlm.nih.gov/pmc/articles/PMC2515569/ 14
http://www.ncbi.nlm.nih.gov/pmc/articles/PMC314438/ 27
http://www.ncbi.nlm.nih.gov/pubmed/?term=contribution+of+cytotoxic+chemotherpay+to+5+year+survival+in+adult+malignancies 39
http://www.ncbi.nlm.nih.gov/pubmed/14745841 29
http://www.ncbi.nlm.nih.gov/pubmed/16136033 35
http://www.ncbi.nlm.nih.gov/pubmed/16870085 40
http://www.ncbi.nlm.nih.gov/pubmed/17090521 33
http://www.ncbi.nlm.nih.gov/pubmed/18474874 40
http://www.ncbi.nlm.nih.gov/pubmed/19930978 35
http://www.ncbi.nlm.nih.gov/pubmed/19967558 40
http://www.ncbi.nlm.nih.gov/pubmed/20035381 40
http://www.ncbi.nlm.nih.gov/pubmed/20097718 40
http://www.ncbi.nlm.nih.gov/pubmed/20399042 40
http://www.ncbi.nlm.nih.gov/pubmed/20429308 40
http://www.ncbi.nlm.nih.gov/pubmed/20565864 33
http://www.ncbi.nlm.nih.gov/pubmed/20582702 35
http://www.ncbi.nlm.nih.gov/pubmed/2068666 33
http://www.ncbi.nlm.nih.gov/pubmed/21720992 36
http://www.ornishspectrum.com/proven-program/the-research/ 18
http://www.pbs.org/wgbh/pages/frontline/shows/meat/safe/overview.html ..22
http://www.preventcancer.com/publications/pdf/Interview%20%20June%2003.htm 36, 41
http://www.slv.se/upload/heatox/documents/D62_final_project_leaflet.pdf...22
http://www.usda.gov/factbook/chapter2.pdf 20

CHAPTER 2

http://breastcancerconqueror.com/delectable-dishes/ 77
http://breastcancerconqueror.com/raw-almond-bruschetta-crackers/ 67
http://breastcancerconquerorshop.com/product/berkey-water-filter/ 55
http://breastcancerconquerorshop.com/product/broccoli-sprout-powder/.....62, 160, 174, 191
http://breastcancerconquerorshop.com/product/one-world-whey-vanilla-1-lb/ 71, 160

CHAPTER 3

CHAPTER 4

http://amzn.com/1570629552 115
http://amzn.com/B00898JLS2 117
http://breastcancerconqueror.com/7-ways-melatonin-acts-as-a-breast-cancer-inhibitor/ 124
http://breastcancerconqueror.com/how-to-balance-hormones/ 119
http://breastcancerconqueror.com/store/products/complete-hormones-urinalysis/ 120
http://breastcancerconqueror.com/store/products/comprehensive-plus-panel/ 120
http://breastcancerconqueror.com/why-spend-1-hour-in-the-gym/ 128
http://breastcancerconquerorshop.com/product/comprehensive-saliva-plus-panel/ 118
http://breastcancerconquerorshop.com/product/dim-i3c-healthy-estrogen-support/ 121, 190
http://gongsoundhealing.com/sound-therapy/cancer-sound-healing/ 115
http://jama.jamanetwork.com/article.aspx?articleid=200955 128
http://jama.jamanetwork.com/article.aspx?articleid=200955#REF-JOC50040-4 127
http://onlinelibrary.wiley.com/doi/10.1002/1097-0142(20010915)92:6%2B%3C1689::AID-CNCR1498%3E3.0.CO;2-H/pdf 127
http://summaries.cochrane.org/CD006145/the-effect-of-exercise-on-fatigue-associated-with-cancer 127
http://tulane.edu/news/newwave/121108_blask.cfm 124
http://www.bmj.com/content/321/7274/1424 127
http://www.cancer.gov/cancertopics/factsheet/Therapy/photodynamic 115
http://www.cancer.gov/ncicancerbulletin/062910/page5 126
http://www.chiro.org/research/ABSTRACTS/Immune.shtml 112
http://www.chiro.org/research/ABSTRACTS/Immune_Responses_to_Spinal_Manipulation.shtml 112
http://www.darksideofsleepingpills.com/ 126
http://www.greenmedinfo.com/affiliate/2929/node/102238 110
http://www.imrs2000.com/pemf-book/#.UxDb_PldV0w 114
http://www.labrix.com/InformationResearch 118
http://www.macmillan.org.uk/Cancerinformation/Livingwithandaftercancer/Physicalactivity/Physicalactivityandcancer/Benefits.aspx 128
http://www.maturitas.org/article/S0378-5122%2808%2900204-1/abstract 121

http://www.maximizedliving.com/ 112
http://www.maximizedliving.com/Home/FindaDoctor.aspx 112
http://www.medicalnewstoday.com/releases/31689.php 114
http://www.medscape.org/viewarticle/502825 123
http://www.ncbi.nlm.nih.gov/pmc/articles/PMC1297510/ 116, 117
http://www.ncbi.nlm.nih.gov/pmc/articles/PMC284388/ 112
http://www.ncbi.nlm.nih.gov/pubmed/12946654?dopt=Abstract 123
http://www.ncbi.nlm.nih.gov/pubmed/15947468 110
http://www.ncbi.nlm.nih.gov/pubmed/20042408 123
http://www.ncbi.nlm.nih.gov/pubmed/20607384 126
http://www.ncbi.nlm.nih.gov/pubmed/20864719 126
http://www.ncbi.nlm.nih.gov/pubmed/22459520 113
http://www.ncbi.nlm.nih.gov/pubmed/22830442 126
http://www.ncbi.nlm.nih.gov/pubmed/22851666 127
http://www.ncbi.nlm.nih.gov/pubmed/23788992 127
http://www.ncbi.nlm.nih.gov/pubmed/23955127 115
http://www.ncbi.nlm.nih.gov/pubmed/24039828 114
http://www.ncbi.nlm.nih.gov/pubmed/2702580 119
http://www.ncbi.nlm.nih.gov/pubmed/6204761 110
http://www.ncbi.nlm.nih.gov/pubmed/9369454 119
http://www.nccaom.org/ 113
http://www.nih.gov/researchmatters/december2011/12052011light.htm 116
http://www.psychosomaticmedicine.org/content/60/1/48.abstract 123
http://www.sonophotodynamictherapy.com/index.html 116
http://www.sonophotodynamictherapy.com/sonophotodynamictherapy_therapy.html 116
http://www.tahomaclinic.com/ 120
http://www.virginiahopkinstestkits.com/bioidenticalbreastcancer.html 121
Murray DR, Irwin M, Reardon CA, et al. "Sympathetic and immune interactions during dynamic exercise. Mediation via a beta 2 - adrenergic-dependent mechanism." Circulation 1992 86(1): 203 111
Pero R. "Medical Researcher Excited By CBSRF Project Results." The Chiropractic Journal, August 1989; 32 111

CHAPTER 5

http://amzn.com/0553280333 .... 134, 142
http://breastcancerconqueror.com/videos/ 148

http://candacepert.com/ ... 146, 148
http://dictionary.reference.com/browse/happy ... 142
http://phys.org/news63293074.html ... 145
http://science.howstuffworks.com/life/exercise-happiness2.htm ... 145
http://science.howstuffworks.com/life/happy-people-live-longer.htm ... 142
http://www.alternative-cancer-care.com/the-cancer-personality.html ... 134
http://www.amazon.com/Love-Medicine-Miracles-Self-Healing-Exceptional-ebook/dp/B005AJQKBO/ref=sr_1_2?s=books&ie=UTF8&qid=1389287206&sr=1-2&keywords=bernie+siegel+books ... 137
http://www.amazon.com/Placebo-Effects-Understanding-mechanisms-disease/dp/0199559120 ... 137
http://www.ariseindiaforum.org/nurse-reveals-the-top-5-regrets-people-make-on-their-deathbed/ ... 148
http://www.ncbi.nlm.nih.gov/pubmed/11374751 ... 143
http://www.ncbi.nlm.nih.gov/pubmed/16262767 ... 142
Pierre Kissel and Dominique Barrucand, Placebos et Effet Placebo en Médecine (Paris: Masson, 1964) ... 137

CHAPTER 6

http://breastcancerconqueror.com/bpa-and-breast-cancer/ ... 155
http://breastcancerconqueror.com/is-your-root-canal-increasing-your-risk-for-breast-cancer/ ... 156
http://breastcancerconquerorshop.com/product/chlorella/ ... 160
http://dentalwellness4u.com/index.html ... 153
http://orthomolecular.org/library/jom/1983/pdf/1983-v12n03-p184.pdf ... 154
http://terfinfo.com/ ... 156
http://www.biocomplabs.com/index.html ... 152
http://www.ccrlab.com/ ... 152
http://www.isisboston.com/assets/PDF-Files/Tooth-Organ-Chart.pdf ... 157, 161
http://www.issels.com/history.aspx#sthash.If6QomJa.dpbs ... 156
http://www.ncbi.nlm.nih.gov/pubmed/12088666 ... 156
http://www.ncbi.nlm.nih.gov/pubmed/15712295 ... 154
http://www.ncbi.nlm.nih.gov/pubmed/16489580 ... 154
http://www.ncbi.nlm.nih.gov/pubmed/16804515 ... 154
http://www.ncbi.nlm.nih.gov/pubmed/22422990 ... 154
http://www.new-cancer-treatments.org/Articles/RootCanals.html ... 156

https://www.jstage.jst.go.jp/result?cdjournal=jts&item1=4&word1=
methyl+
mercury+and+chlorella 160

CHAPTER 7

Finley JW, Bogardus, GM. Breast Cancer and Thyroid Disease Quart. Review Surg Obstet Gyn 17:139-147, 1960 198
http://amzn.com/B0036USKX0 217
http://ascendingstarseed.wordpress.com/2013/11/07/spain-study-confirms-hemp-oil-cures-cancer-without-side-effects/ 183
http://blogs.ocweekly.com/navelgazing/2013/04/bay_area_researchers_claim_can.php 182
http://breastcancerconqueror.com/about-dr-v/contact/ 182
http://breastcancerconqueror.com/have-you-heard-of-poly-mva/ 186
http://breastcancerconqueror.com/spirulina-a-powerful-anti-cancer-super-food/ 186
http://breastcancerconquerorshop.com/?s=whey&post_type=product 195
http://breastcancerconquerorshop.com/product/beta-13-d-glucan/ 188
http://breastcancerconquerorshop.com/product/brevail-2/ 197
http://breastcancerconquerorshop.com/product/cancer-x-spirulina-1-lb-powder/ 187
http://breastcancerconquerorshop.com/product/chaga-750-ct/ 188
http://breastcancerconquerorshop.com/product/chaga-tea-1lb/ 188
http://breastcancerconquerorshop.com/product/healthy-girls-breast-oil/ 219
http://breastcancerconquerorshop.com/product/liposomal-magnesium-original-flavor-10-oz/ 199
http://breastcancerconquerorshop.com/product/optimal-magnesium/ 199
http://breastcancerconquerorshop.com/product/procella/ 211
http://breastcancerconquerorshop.com/product/vitamin-d-blood-drop-test/ 204, 239
http://breastcancerconquerorshop.com/product-category/essential-1-let-food-be-your-medicine/ 192
http://breastcancerconquerorshop.com/product-category/homeopathics/ 190
http://breastcancerconquerorshop.com/product-category/perfect-balance/ . 185
http://cancerx.org/Enzyme%20NOVAK-TRNKA.pdf 172
http://dixiebotanicals.com/products/salvation-balm/ 218
http://drsircus.com/ 199

http://www.ncbi.nlm.nih.gov/pmc/articles/PMC2996866/ 170
http://www.ncbi.nlm.nih.gov/pmc/articles/PMC3673330/ 171
http://www.ncbi.nlm.nih.gov/pubmed/?term=pau+d%27arco++breast+cancer 190
http://www.ncbi.nlm.nih.gov/pubmed/?term=PMC314438 198
http://www.ncbi.nlm.nih.gov/pubmed/?term=una+de+gato+breast+cancer 190
http://www.ncbi.nlm.nih.gov/pubmed/?term=vitamin+d3+breast+cancer 205
http://www.ncbi.nlm.nih.gov/pubmed/10362108 208
http://www.ncbi.nlm.nih.gov/pubmed/11496322 181
http://www.ncbi.nlm.nih.gov/pubmed/12181239 216
http://www.ncbi.nlm.nih.gov/pubmed/12537959 195, 215
http://www.ncbi.nlm.nih.gov/pubmed/12588701 181
http://www.ncbi.nlm.nih.gov/pubmed/12840226 194
http://www.ncbi.nlm.nih.gov/pubmed/14518774 213
http://www.ncbi.nlm.nih.gov/pubmed/14687793 196
http://www.ncbi.nlm.nih.gov/pubmed/15221974 196
http://www.ncbi.nlm.nih.gov/pubmed/15650394 195
http://www.ncbi.nlm.nih.gov/pubmed/15661811 194
http://www.ncbi.nlm.nih.gov/pubmed/16025225 198
http://www.ncbi.nlm.nih.gov/pubmed/16392670 183
http://www.ncbi.nlm.nih.gov/pubmed/16488130 194
http://www.ncbi.nlm.nih.gov/pubmed/16651453 194
http://www.ncbi.nlm.nih.gov/pubmed/16880611 174
http://www.ncbi.nlm.nih.gov/pubmed/16905640 177
http://www.ncbi.nlm.nih.gov/pubmed/16969125 191
http://www.ncbi.nlm.nih.gov/pubmed/17161824 188
http://www.ncbi.nlm.nih.gov/pubmed/17430183 215
http://www.ncbi.nlm.nih.gov/pubmed/17569208 178
http://www.ncbi.nlm.nih.gov/pubmed/17723168 177
http://www.ncbi.nlm.nih.gov/pubmed/17893836 173
http://www.ncbi.nlm.nih.gov/pubmed/17956159 218
http://www.ncbi.nlm.nih.gov/pubmed/18025276 183
http://www.ncbi.nlm.nih.gov/pubmed/18288407 190
http://www.ncbi.nlm.nih.gov/pubmed/18461293 192
http://www.ncbi.nlm.nih.gov/pubmed/19053851 188
http://www.ncbi.nlm.nih.gov/pubmed/19250217 178
http://www.ncbi.nlm.nih.gov/pubmed/19423769 192

http://www.ncbi.nlm.nih.gov/pubmed/19522736 200
http://www.ncbi.nlm.nih.gov/pubmed/19703194 178
http://www.ncbi.nlm.nih.gov/pubmed/19724995 190
http://www.ncbi.nlm.nih.gov/pubmed/19809577 178
http://www.ncbi.nlm.nih.gov/pubmed/19908170 178
http://www.ncbi.nlm.nih.gov/pubmed/20152024 191
http://www.ncbi.nlm.nih.gov/pubmed/20155630 206
http://www.ncbi.nlm.nih.gov/pubmed/20193099 192
http://www.ncbi.nlm.nih.gov/pubmed/20550747 192
http://www.ncbi.nlm.nih.gov/pubmed/20607061 189
http://www.ncbi.nlm.nih.gov/pubmed/20646066 178
http://www.ncbi.nlm.nih.gov/pubmed/20859676 183
http://www.ncbi.nlm.nih.gov/pubmed/21097717 196
http://www.ncbi.nlm.nih.gov/pubmed/21269259 212
http://www.ncbi.nlm.nih.gov/pubmed/21428708 212
http://www.ncbi.nlm.nih.gov/pubmed/21489580 191
http://www.ncbi.nlm.nih.gov/pubmed/21520988 196
http://www.ncbi.nlm.nih.gov/pubmed/21566064 183
http://www.ncbi.nlm.nih.gov/pubmed/21617865 177
http://www.ncbi.nlm.nih.gov/pubmed/21713389 178
http://www.ncbi.nlm.nih.gov/pubmed/21756879 174
http://www.ncbi.nlm.nih.gov/pubmed/21995112 200
http://www.ncbi.nlm.nih.gov/pubmed/22021693 204
http://www.ncbi.nlm.nih.gov/pubmed/22185819 190
http://www.ncbi.nlm.nih.gov/pubmed/22191568 173
http://www.ncbi.nlm.nih.gov/pubmed/22201894 192
http://www.ncbi.nlm.nih.gov/pubmed/22213287 179
http://www.ncbi.nlm.nih.gov/pubmed/22213291 204
http://www.ncbi.nlm.nih.gov/pubmed/22237979 200
http://www.ncbi.nlm.nih.gov/pubmed/22335196 200
http://www.ncbi.nlm.nih.gov/pubmed/22459208 213
http://www.ncbi.nlm.nih.gov/pubmed/22555283 182
http://www.ncbi.nlm.nih.gov/pubmed/22655458 191
http://www.ncbi.nlm.nih.gov/pubmed/22704445 208
http://www.ncbi.nlm.nih.gov/pubmed/22711009 192
http://www.ncbi.nlm.nih.gov/pubmed/22771646 174
http://www.ncbi.nlm.nih.gov/pubmed/22842186 196

CHAPTER 8

INDEX

B

C

D

E

F

G

H

J

K

L

M

Q

R

T

U

V

W

X

Y

Z

ABOUT THE AUTHOR

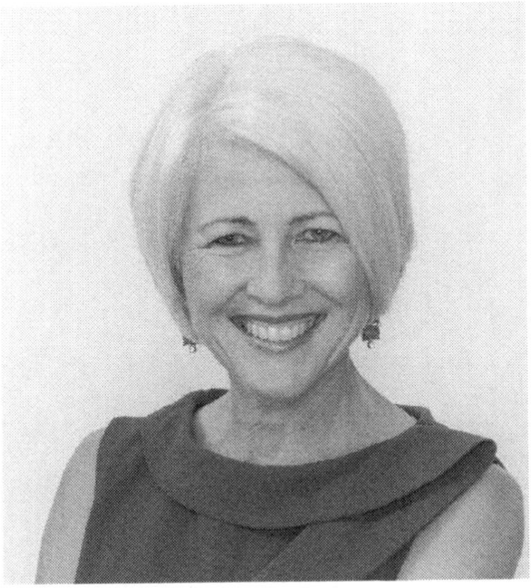

Dr. Véronique Desaulniers-Chomniak, better known as 'Dr. V', has maintained successful practices in the Wellness Field since 1979.

She graduated from Life Chiropractic College in Atlanta, GA, in December of 1979. For the next 20 years, she practiced in middle GA, attracting patients from all over North America and as far as Europe and Africa. The last 10 years of her practice, she focused on Women's Wellness and Breast Cancer prevention.

Because of her passion for health and wellness, Dr. V. undertook extensive studies in various fields of 'Energy Medicine'. Specializing in Bio-Energetics, Meridian Stress Analysis, Homeopathy, Digital Thermography, and Chiropractic, Dr. V. brings a unique approach to Health and Wellness.

After 30 years in active practice, she decided to 'retire' and devote her time to sharing her personal, non-toxic healing journey with Breast Cancer. Her years of experience and research have culminated as 'The 7 Essentials', a step by step coaching program for preventing and healing Breast Cancer Naturally.

When you work with Dr. V., she saves you time, effort, and money by specifically targeting your goals of vibrant health.

Her web site and her personal healing journey have touched the lives of thousands of women around the globe.

Connect with Dr. V online at:

www.BreastCancerConqueror.com

Join the Heal Breast Cancer Naturally Facebook Group:

https://www.facebook.com/groups/1420874398161032/

Join the Facebook Fan Page:

https://www.facebook.com/BreastCancerConqueror

Connect on Twitter:

https://twitter.com/dr_veronique

Connect on LinkedIn:

www.linkedin.com/pub/veronique-desaulniers/12/721/462/

One Last Thing...

If you enjoyed this book or found it useful, I'd be very grateful if you'd post a short review on Amazon. Your support really does make a difference, and I read all the reviews personally so I can get your feedback and make this book and future books even better.

Thank you for your support!

30686054R00169

Made in the USA
Charleston, SC
23 June 2014